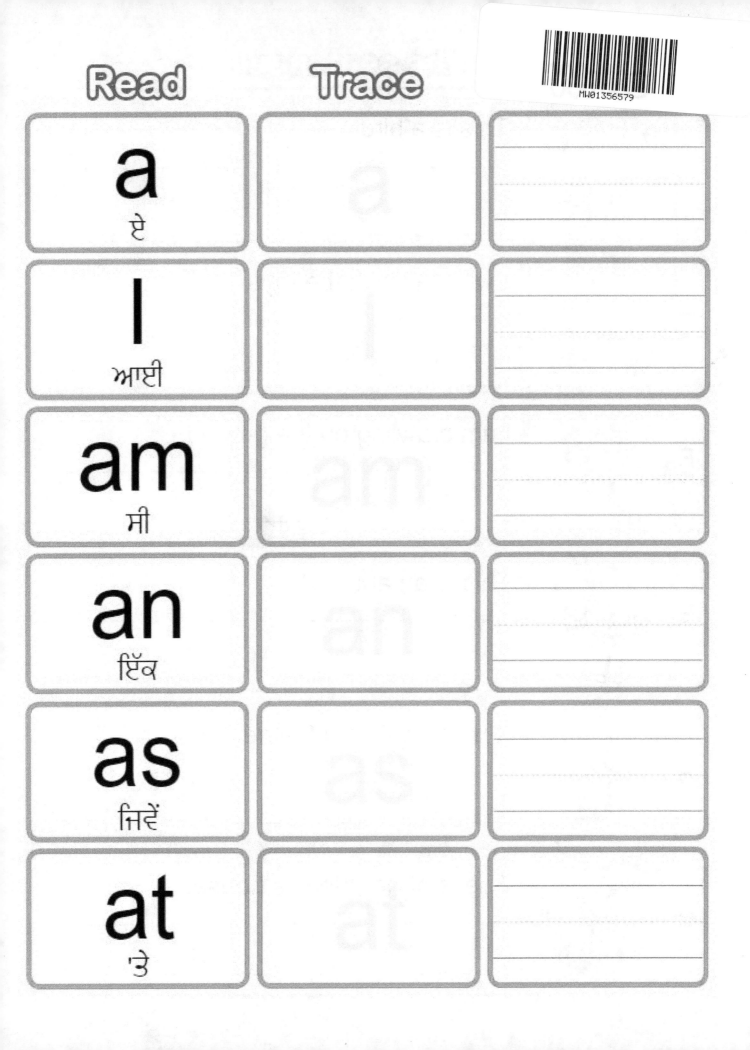

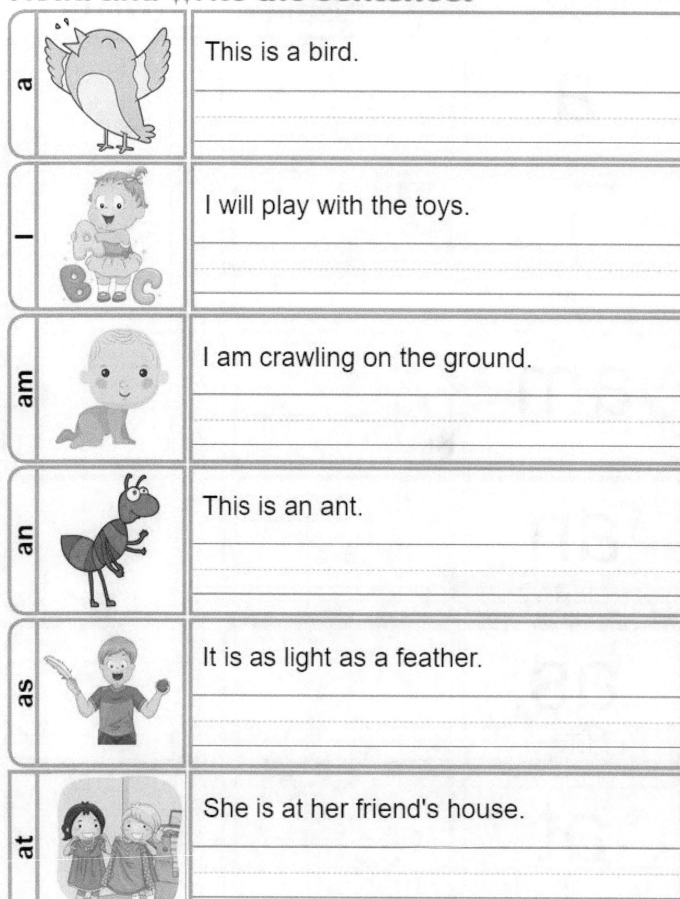

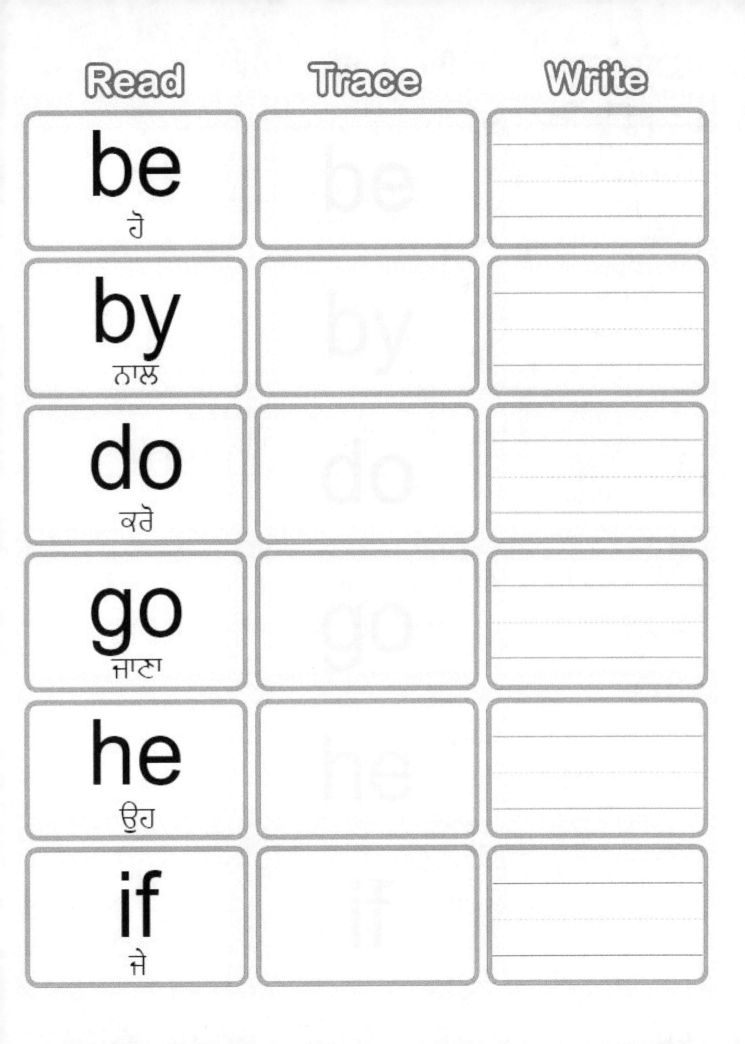

Read and write the sentence!

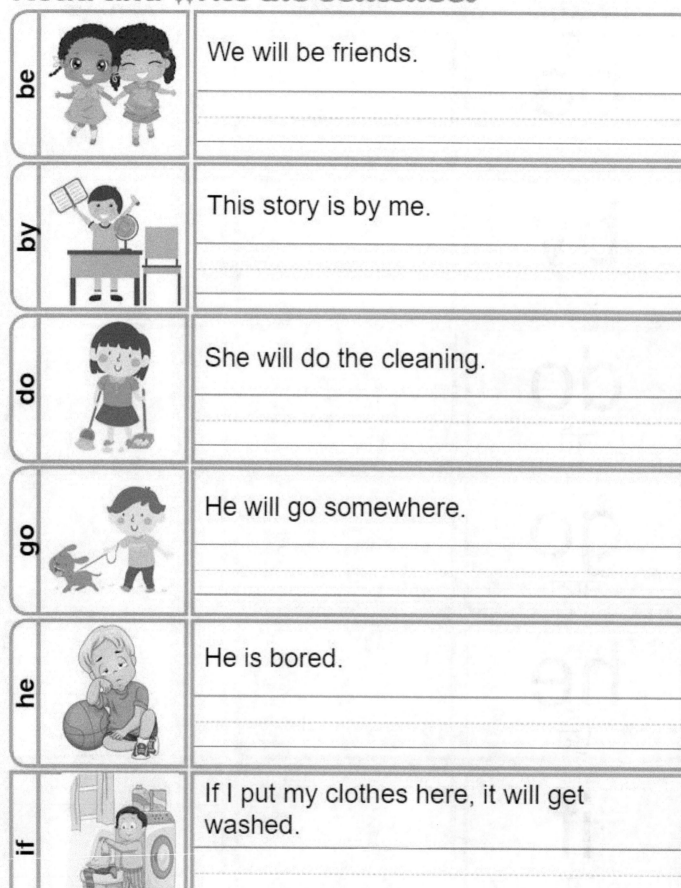

be		We will be friends.
by		This story is by me.
do		She will do the cleaning.
go		He will go somewhere.
he		He is bored.
if		If I put my clothes here, it will get washed.

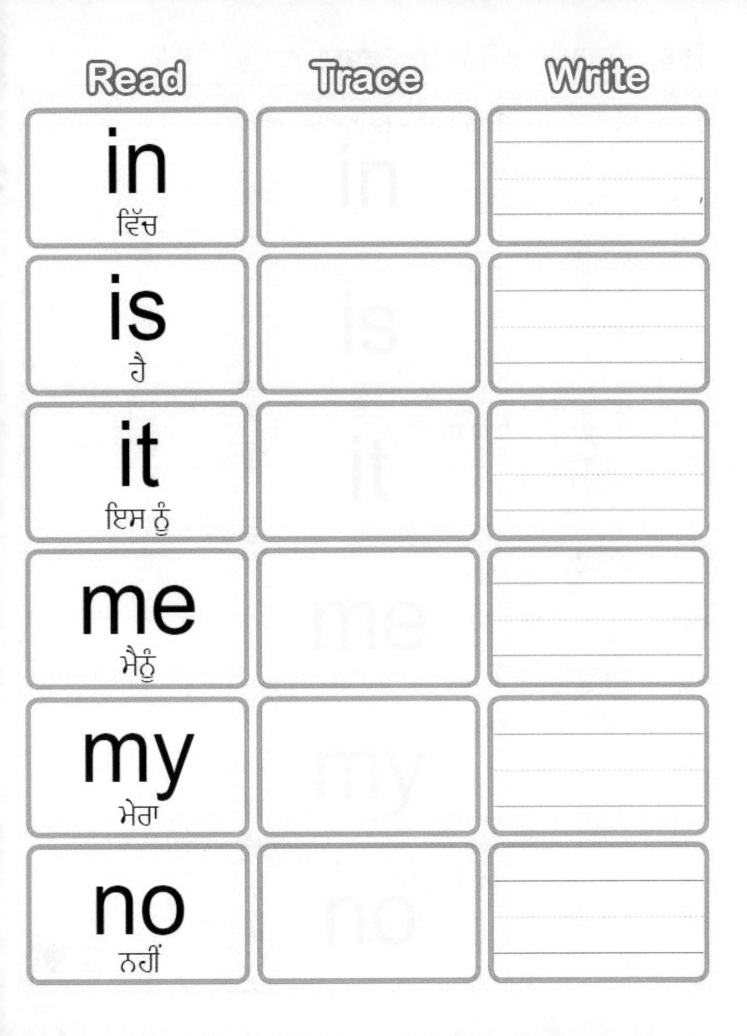

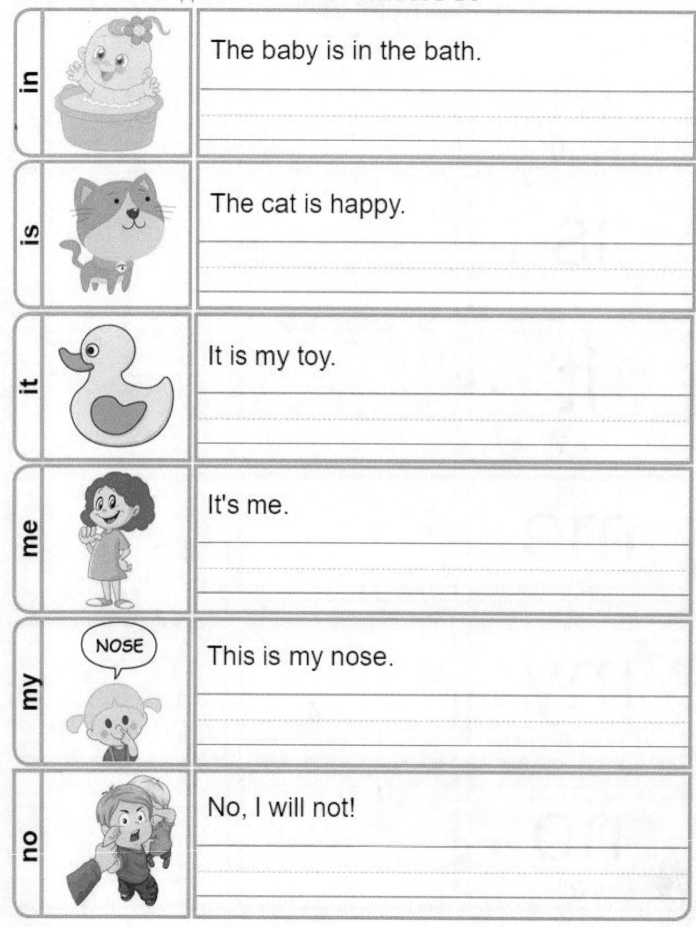

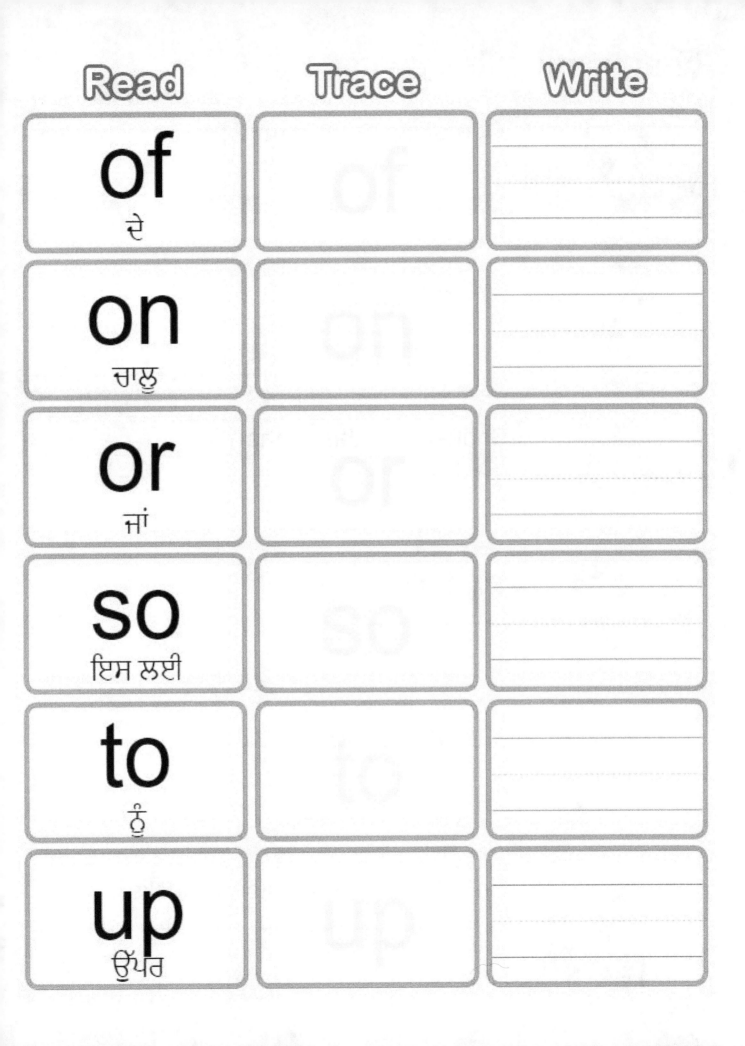

Read and write the sentence!

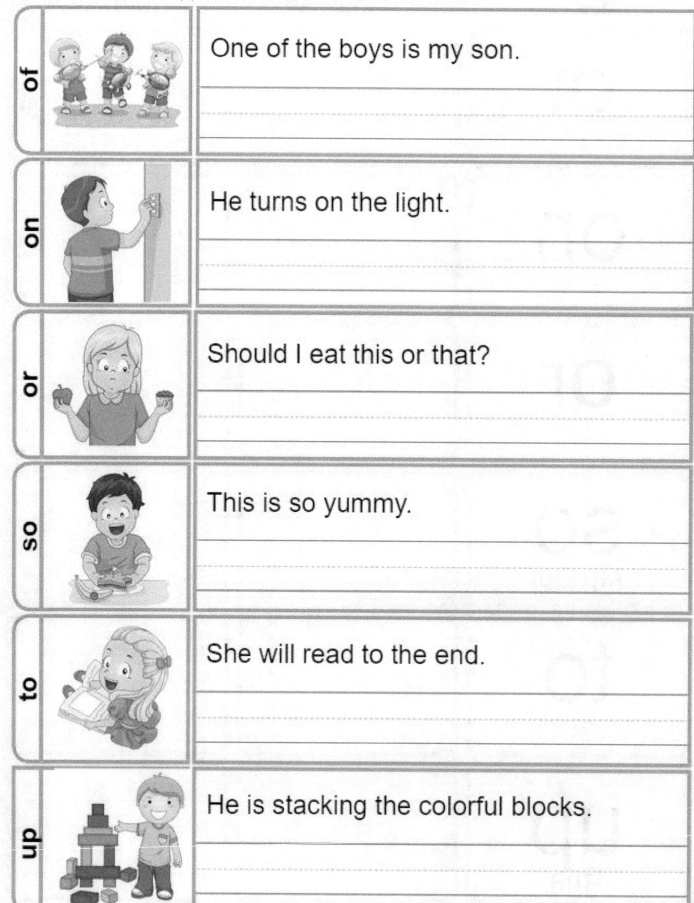

of — One of the boys is my son.

on — He turns on the light.

or — Should I eat this or that?

so — This is so yummy.

to — She will read to the end.

up — He is stacking the colorful blocks.

Read	Trace	Write
us ਸਾਨੂੰ	us	
we ਅਸੀਂ	we	
all ਸਭ	all	
and ਅਤੇ	and	
any ਕੋਈ ਵੀ	any	
are ਹਨ	are	

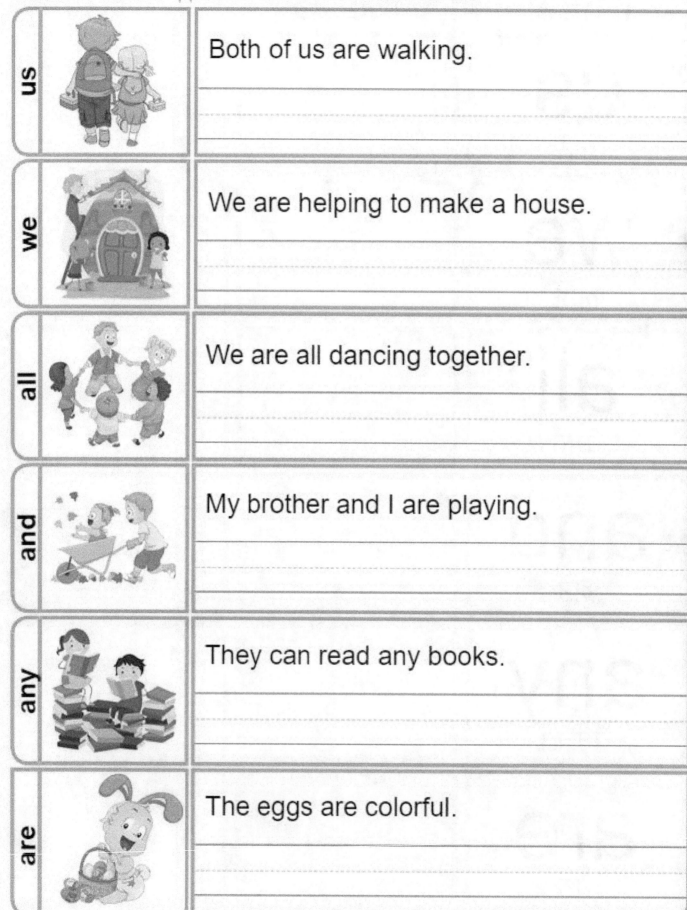

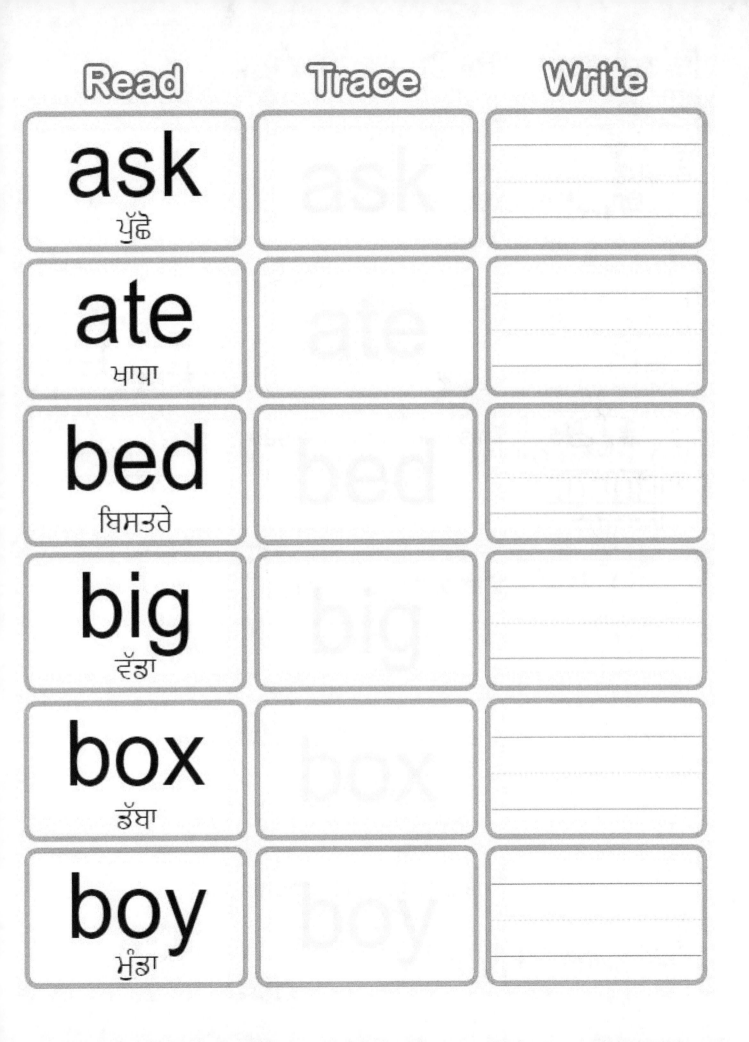

Read and write the sentence!

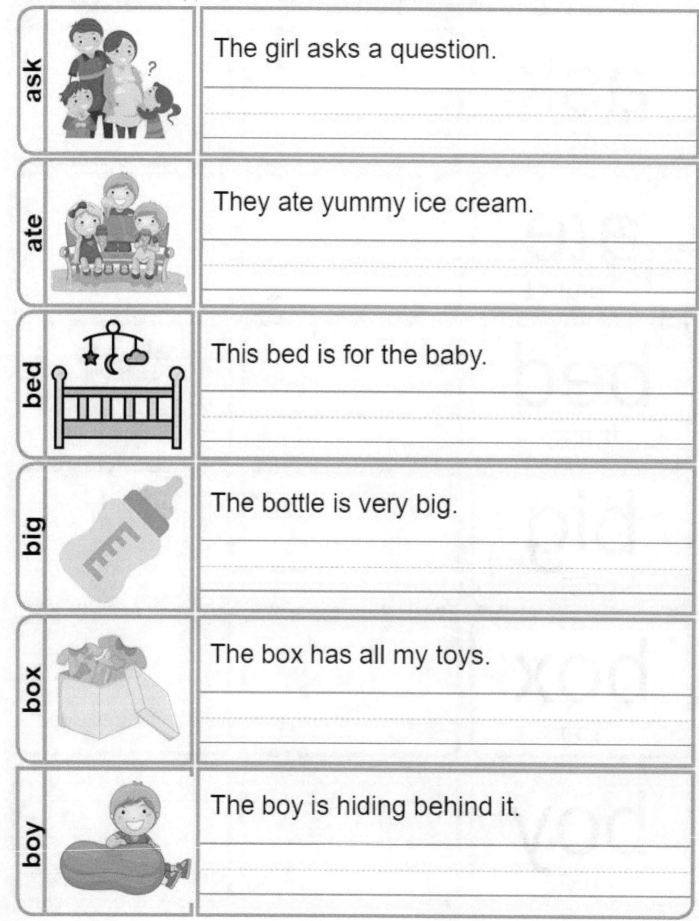

ask		The girl asks a question.
ate		They ate yummy ice cream.
bed		This bed is for the baby.
big		The bottle is very big.
box		The box has all my toys.
boy		The boy is hiding behind it.

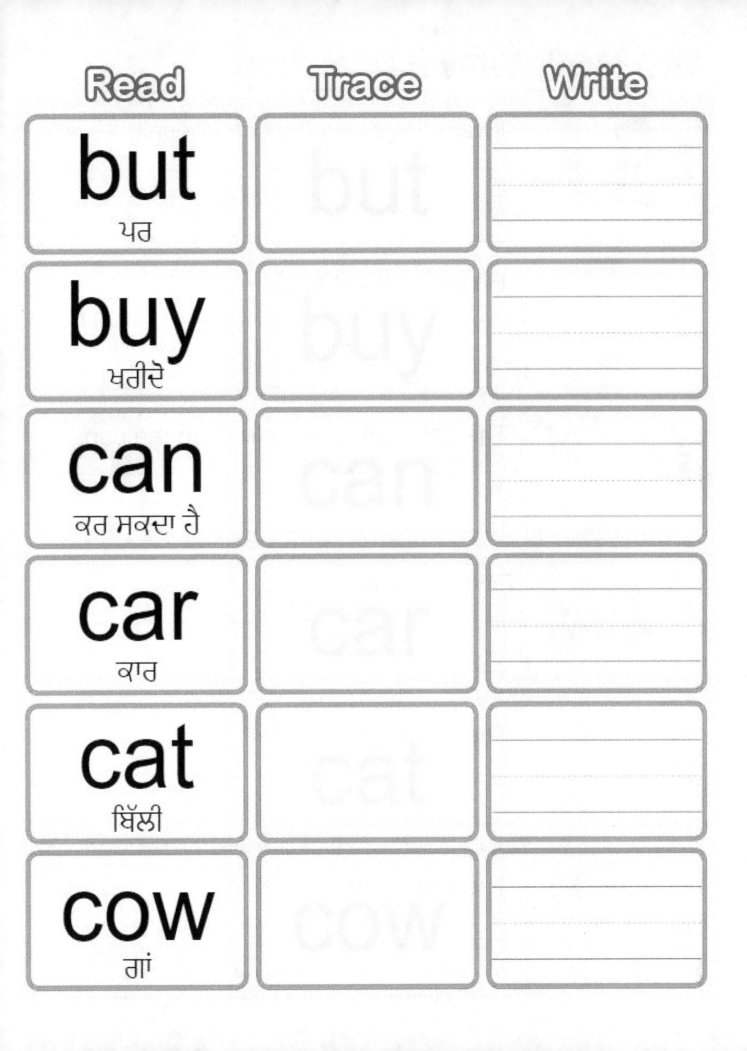

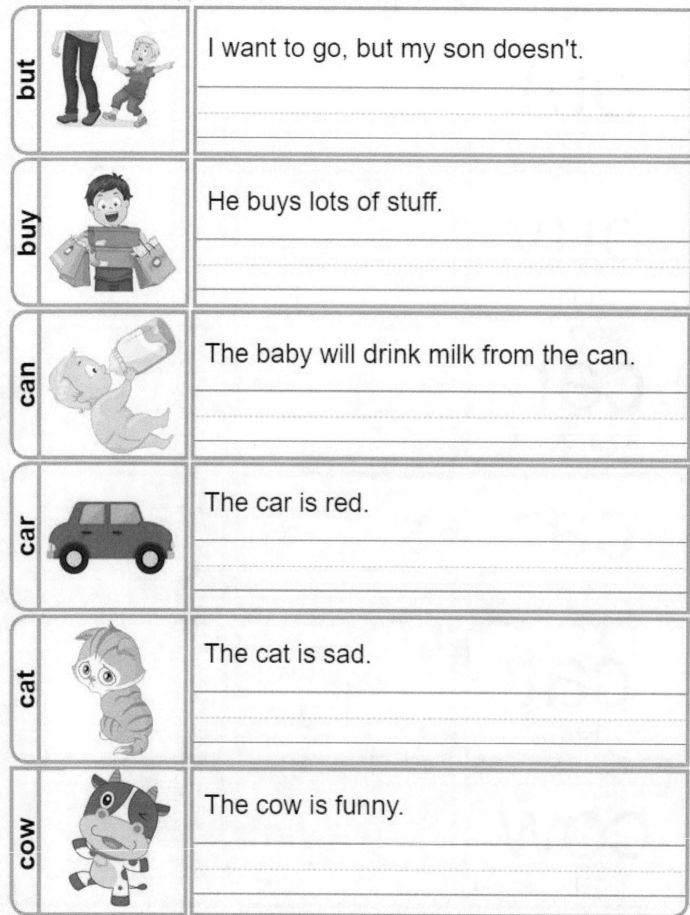

Read	Trace	Write
cut ਕੱਟੋ	cut	
day ਦਿਨ	day	
did ਕੀਤਾ	did	
dog ਕੁੱਤਾ	dog	
eat ਖਾਣਾ	eat	
egg ਆਂਡਾ	egg	

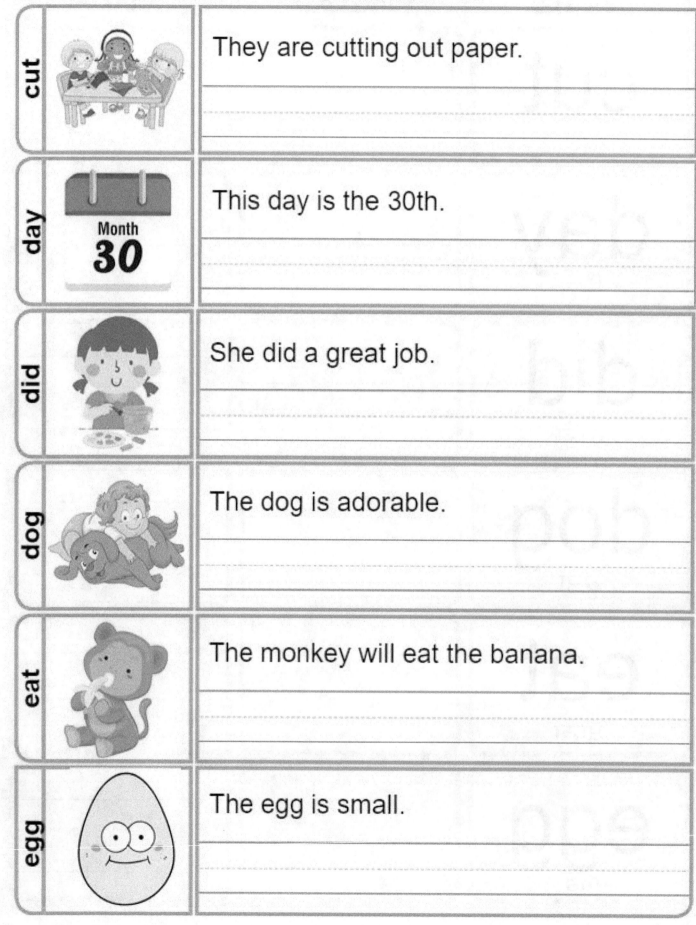

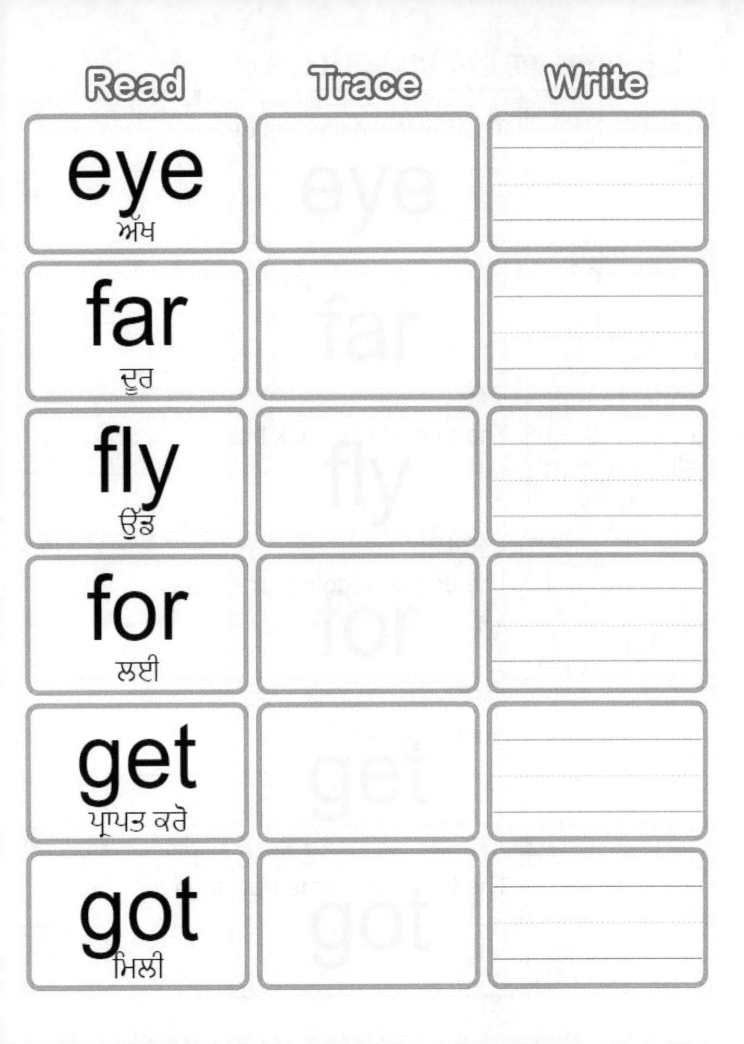

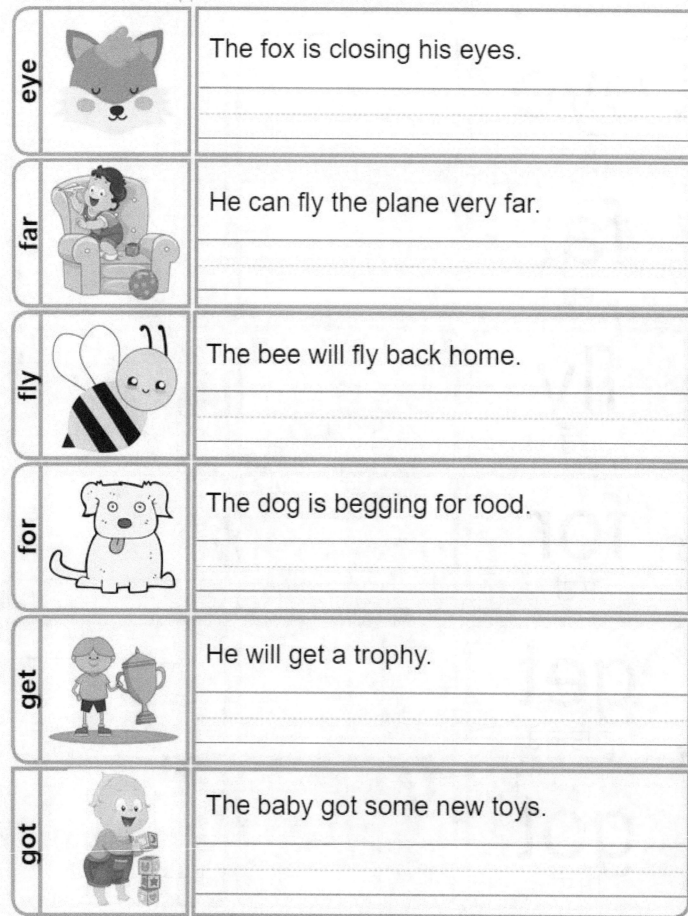

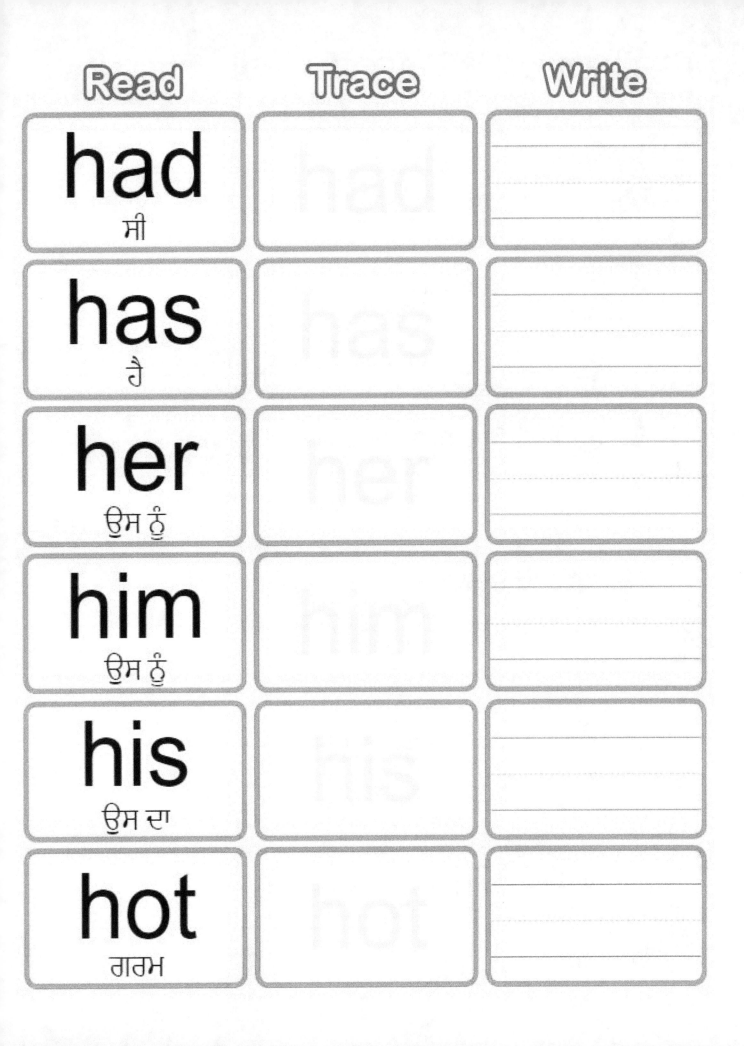

Read and write the sentence!

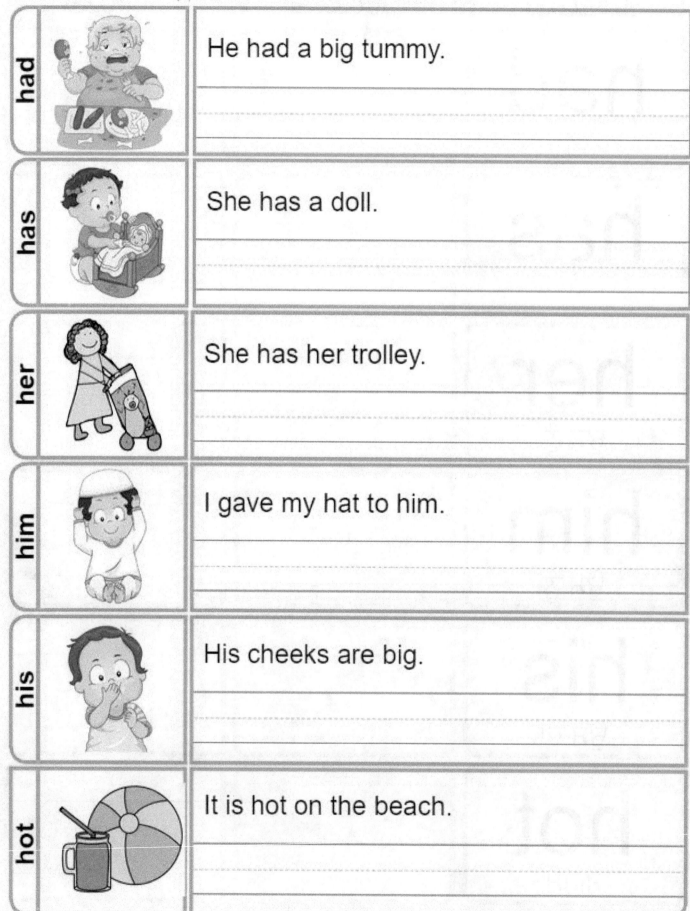

had		He had a big tummy.
has		She has a doll.
her		She has her trolley.
him		I gave my hat to him.
his		His cheeks are big.
hot		It is hot on the beach.

Read	Trace	Write
how ਕਿਵੇਂ	how	
its ਇਸ ਨੂੰ	its	
leg ਲੱਤ	leg	
let ਦਿਉ	let	
man ਆਦਮੀ	man	
may ਹੋ ਸਕਦਾ ਹੈ	may	

Read and write the sentence!

how		How many blocks are there?
its		Its legs are short.
leg		His legs are short.
let		Let me come in!
man		The man is a vet.
may		May I have more?

Read	Trace	Write
men ਆਦਮੀ	men	
new ਨਵਾਂ	new	
not ਨਹੀਂ	not	
now ਹੁਣ	now	
off ਬੰਦ	off	
old ਪੁਰਾਣਾ	old	

Read and write the sentence!

men		The men are mining for gold.
new		She has a new hat.
not		She is not feeling well.
now		Now I am doing my homework.
off		They cut off the paper.
old		You are one year old!

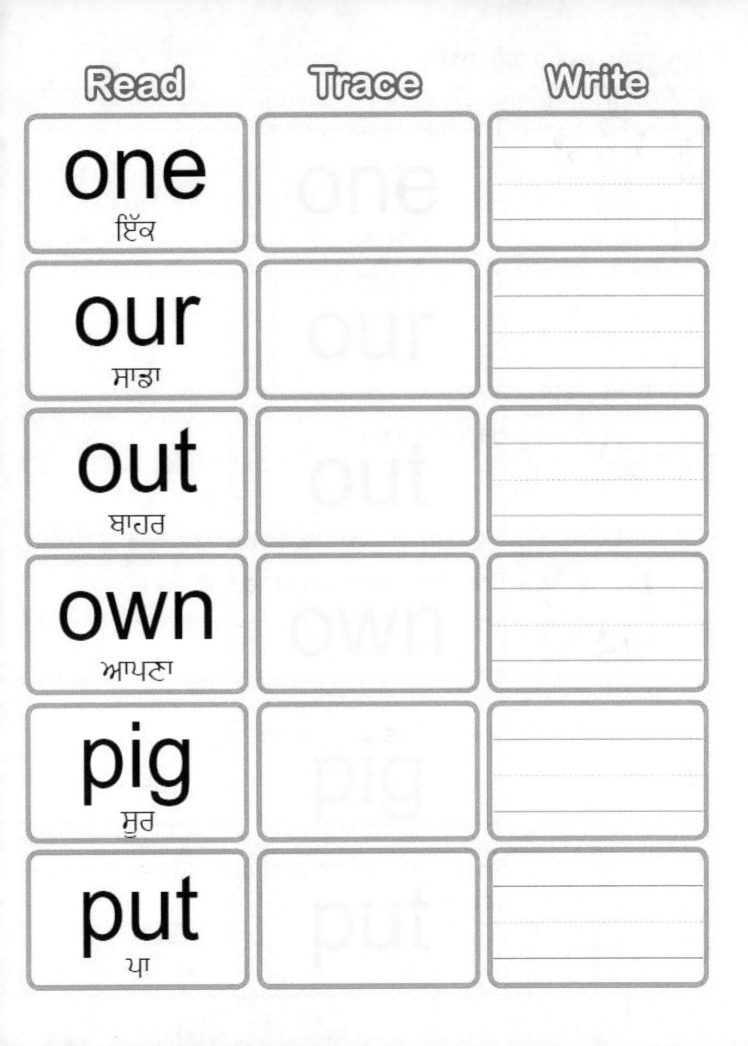

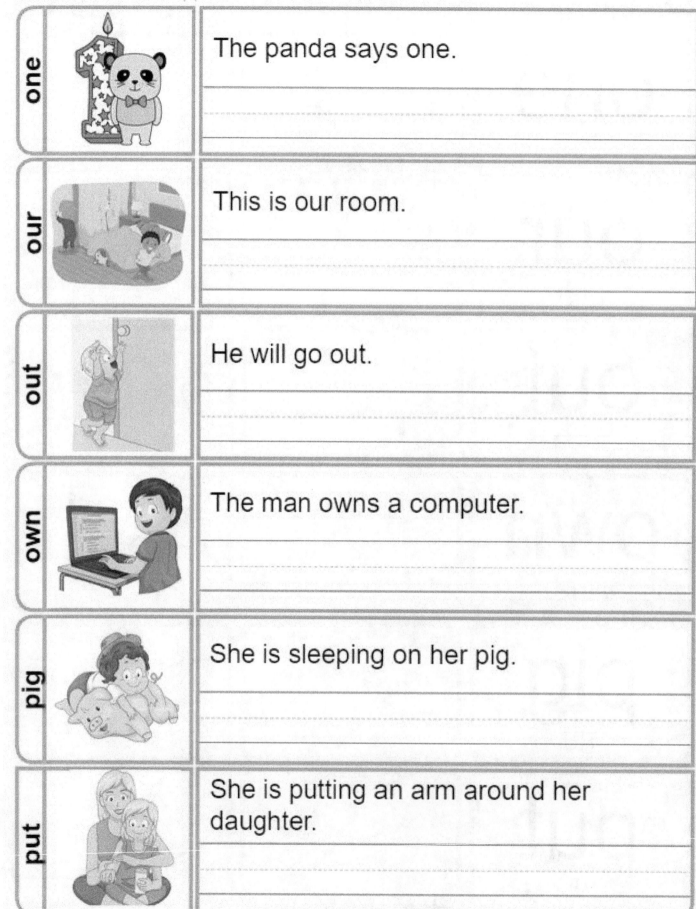

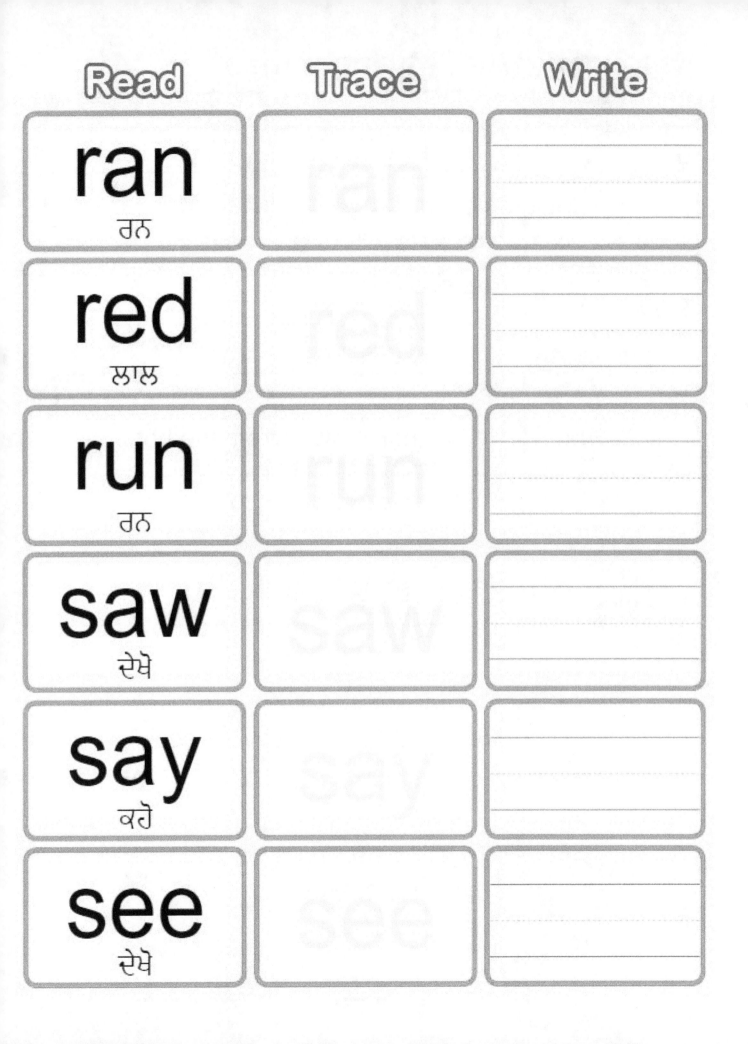

Read and write the sentence!

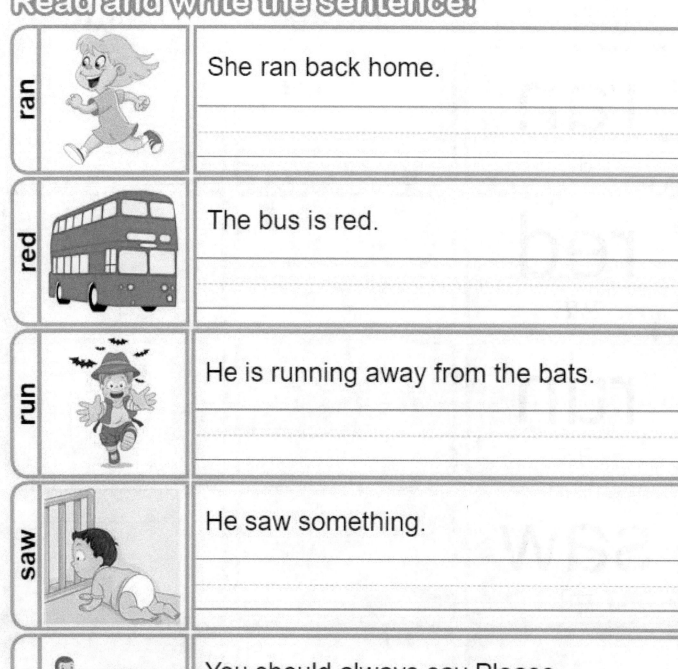

ran		She ran back home.
red		The bus is red.
run		He is running away from the bats.
saw		He saw something.
say		You should always say Please.
see		They see something in the sky.

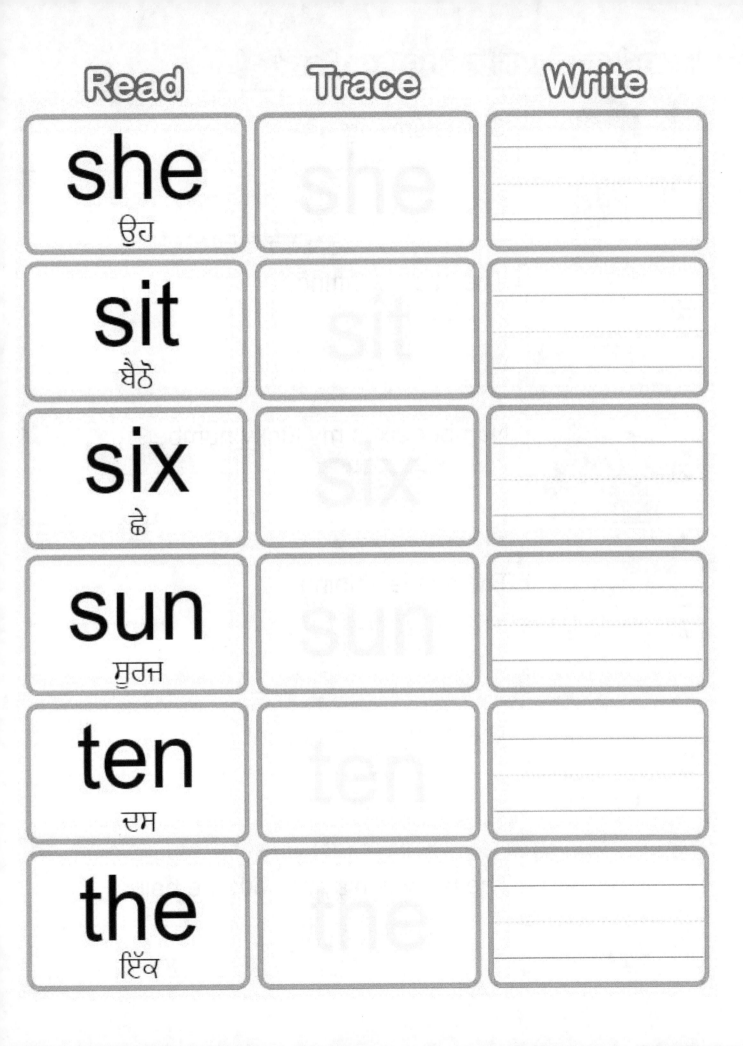

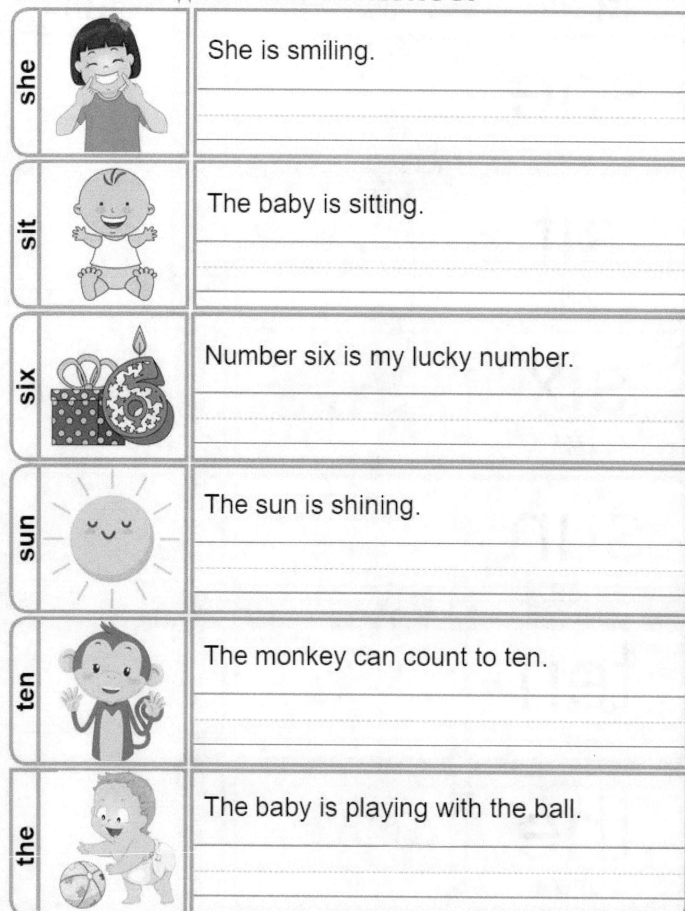

Read	Trace	Write
too ਵੀ	too	
top ਸਿਖਰ	top	
toy ਖਿਡੌਣਾ	toy	
try ਕੋਸ਼ਿਸ਼ ਕਰੋ	try	
two ਦੋ	two	
use ਵਰਤਣ	use	

Read and write the sentence!

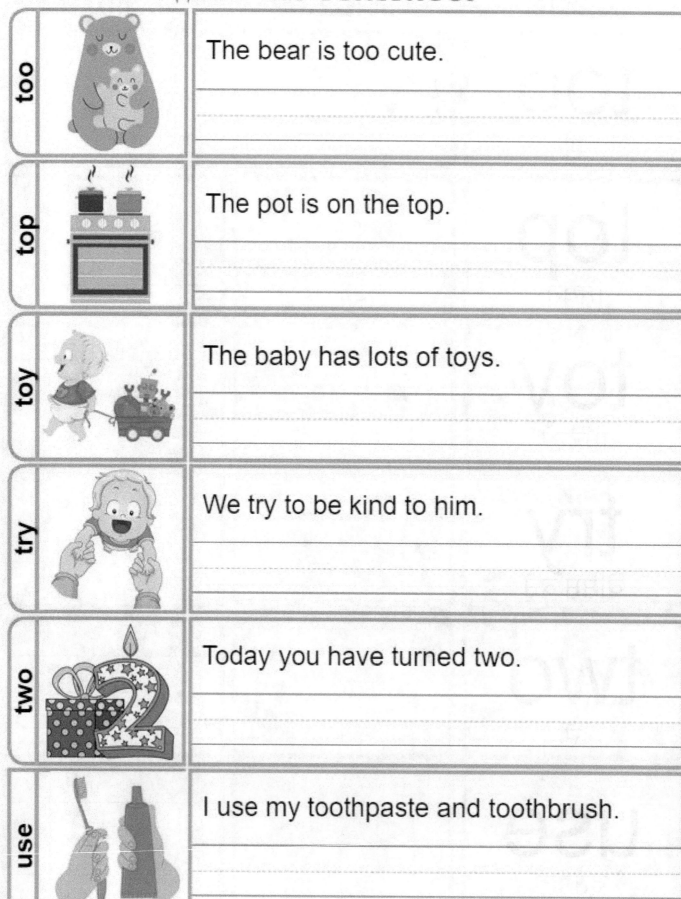

too		The bear is too cute.
top		The pot is on the top.
toy		The baby has lots of toys.
try		We try to be kind to him.
two		Today you have turned two.
use		I use my toothpaste and toothbrush.

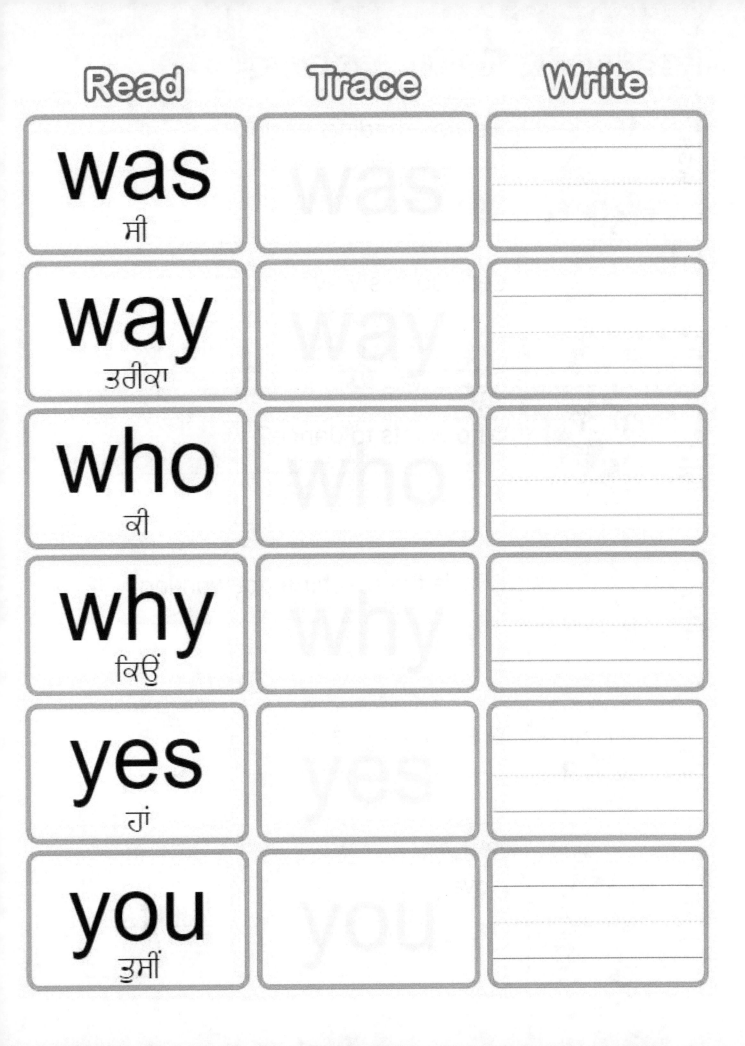

Read and write the sentence!

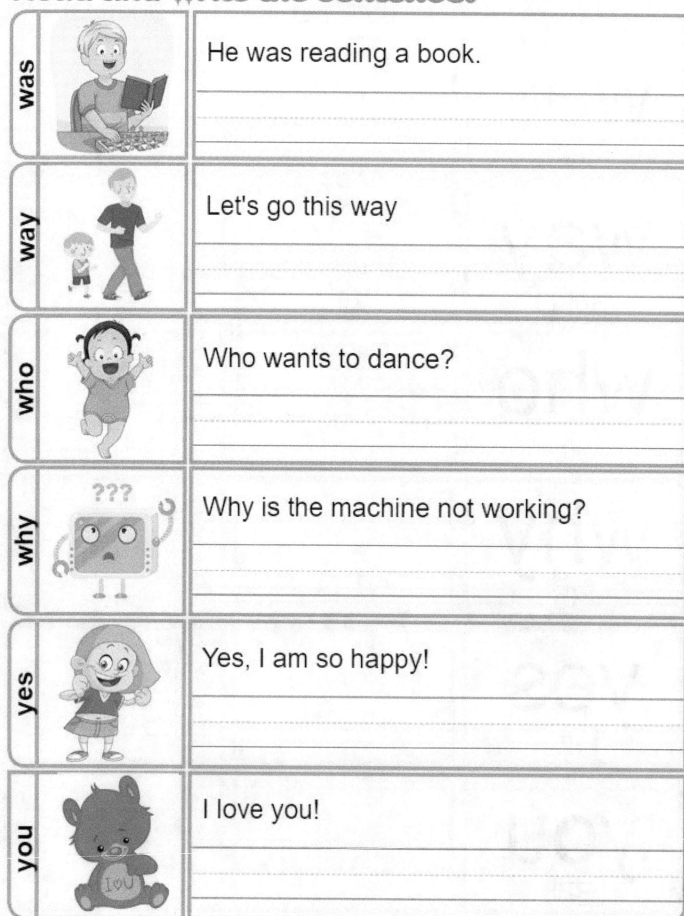

was	He was reading a book.
way	Let's go this way
who	Who wants to dance?
why	Why is the machine not working?
yes	Yes, I am so happy!
you	I love you!

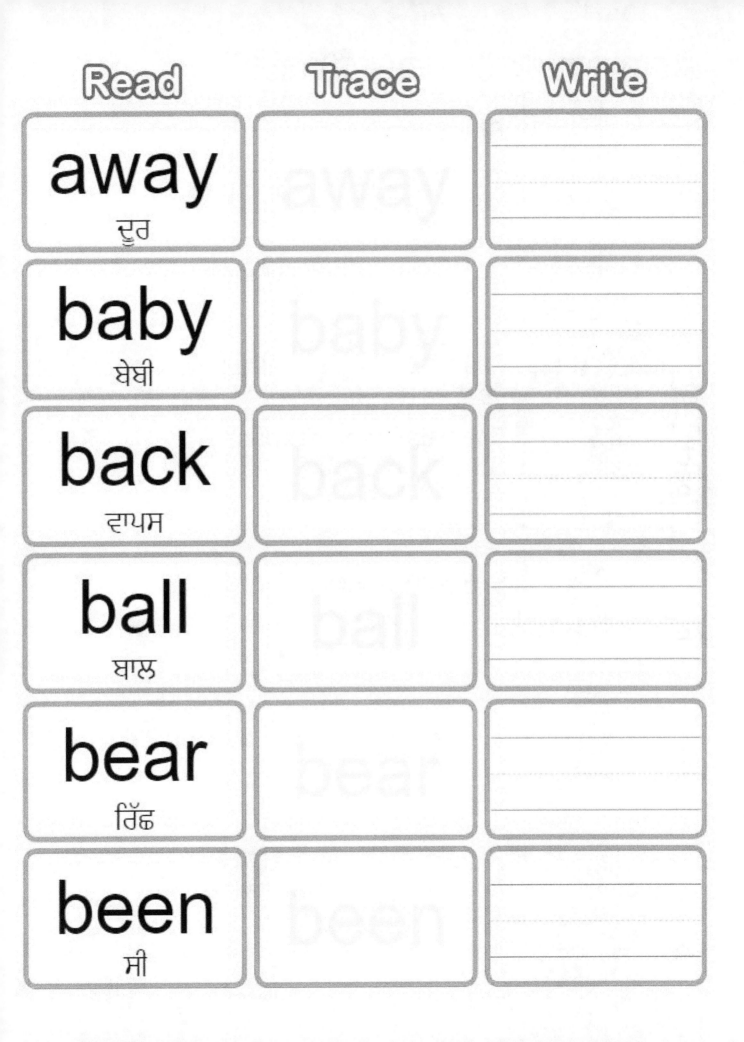

Read and write the sentence!

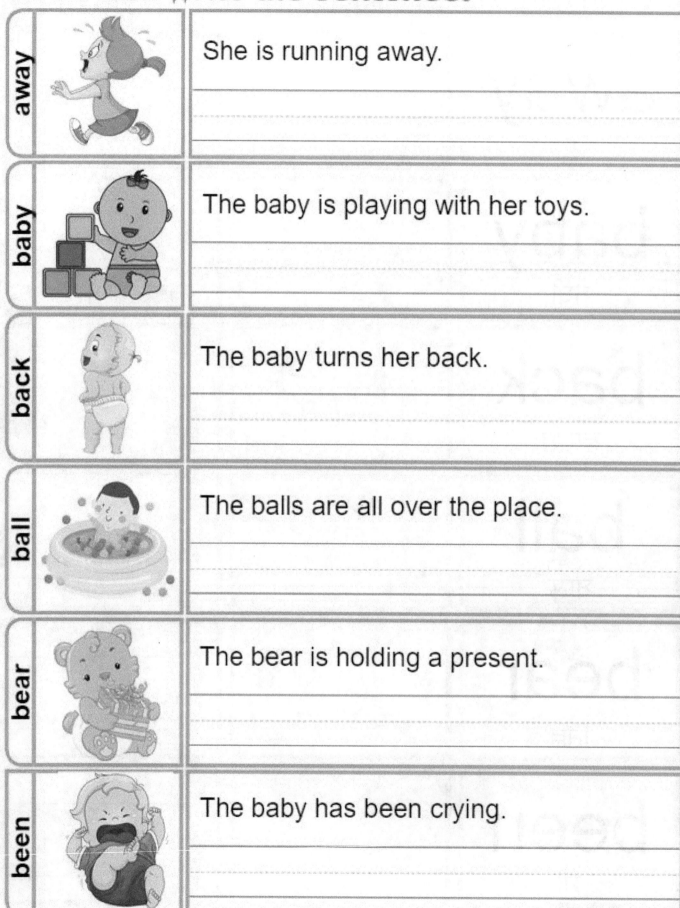

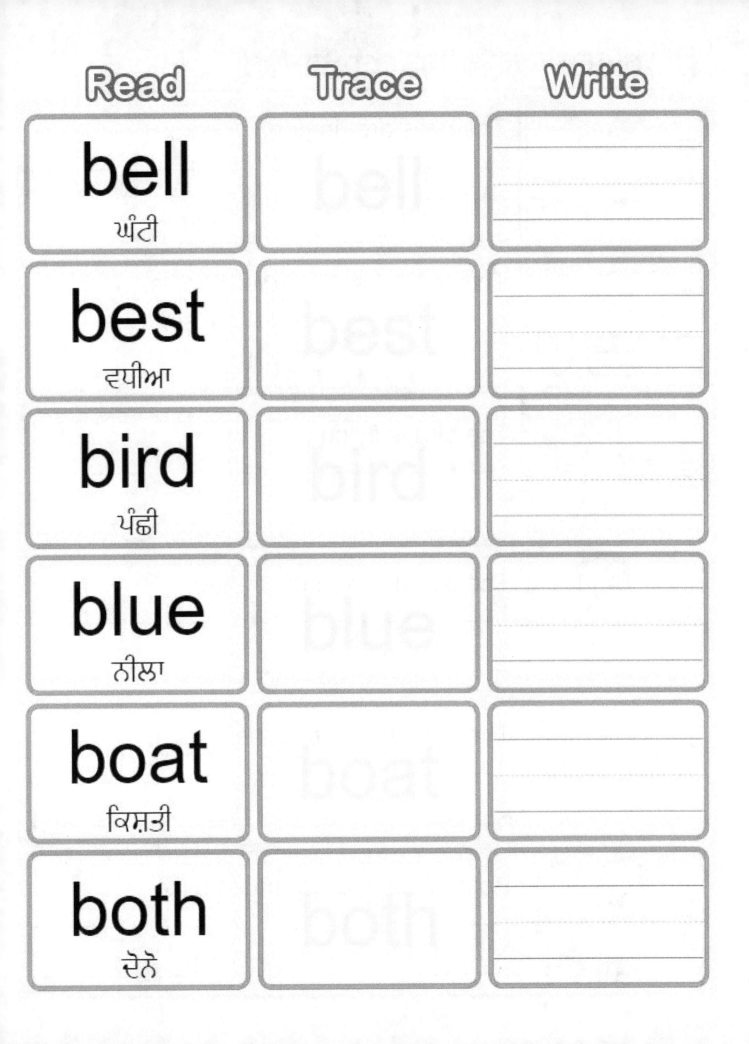

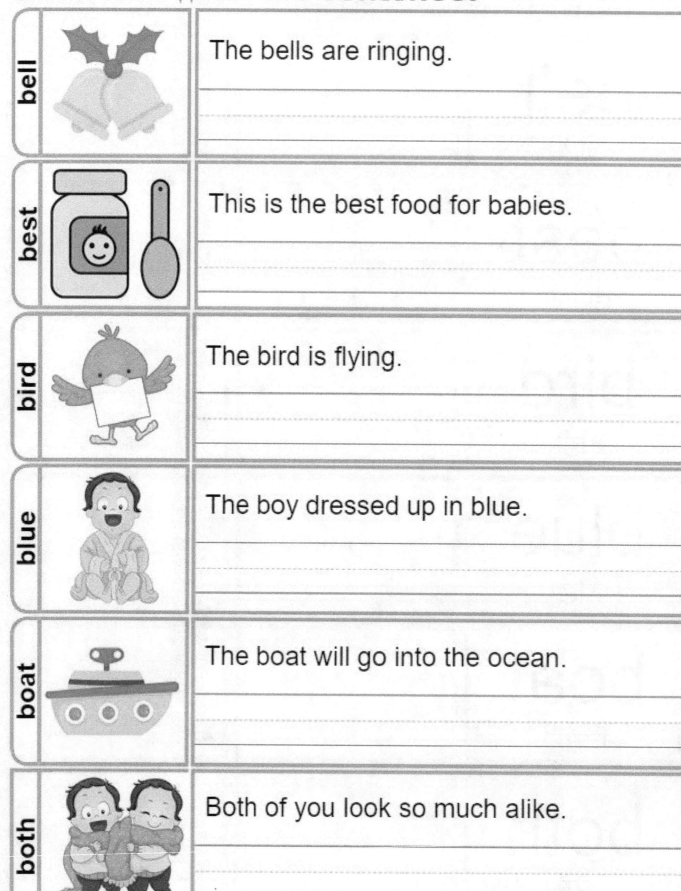

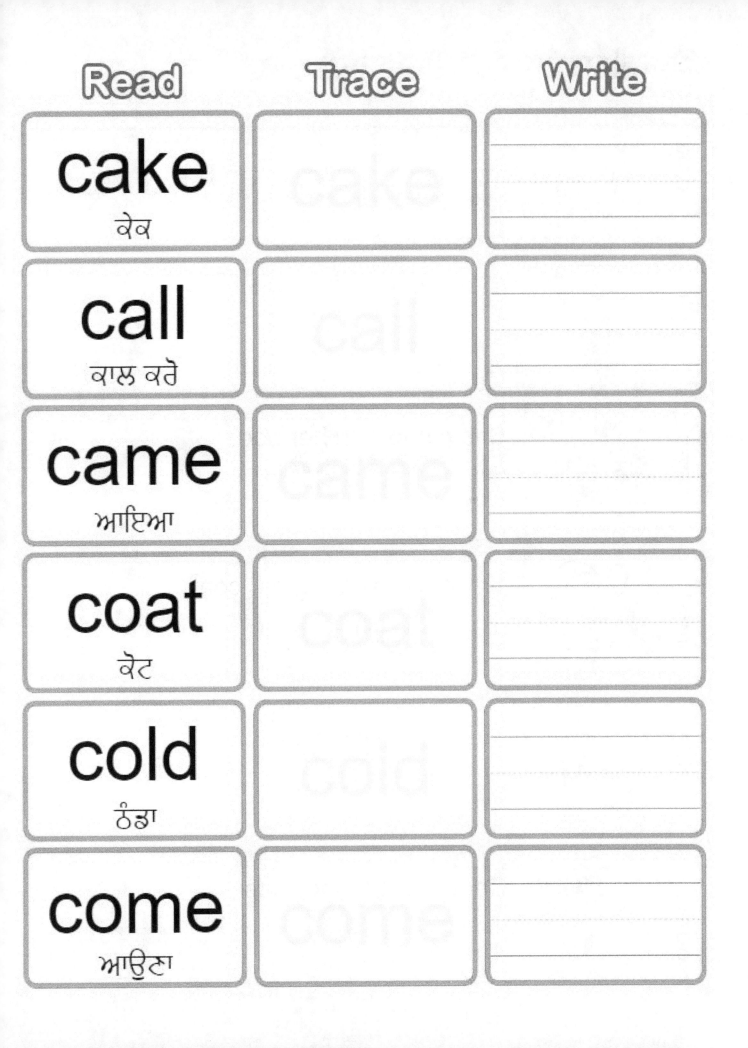

Read and write the sentence!

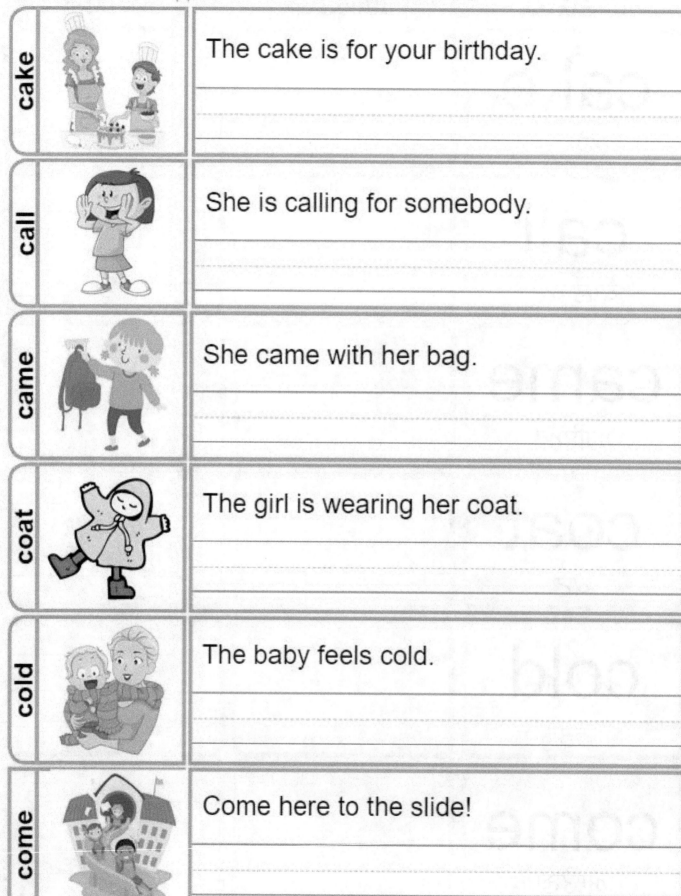

Read	Trace	Write
corn ਮਕਈ	corn	
does ਕਰਦਾ ਹੈ	does	
doll ਗੁੱਡੀ	doll	
done ਕੀਤਾ	done	
door ਦਰਵਾਜ਼ਾ	door	
down ਥੱਲੇ, ਹੇਠਾਂ, ਨੀਂਵਾ	down	

Read and write the sentence!

corn		The corn tastes good.
does		Does that thing taste bad?
doll		She is hugging her doll.
done		I've done reading my book.
door		They open the door.
down		The boy turns his head down.

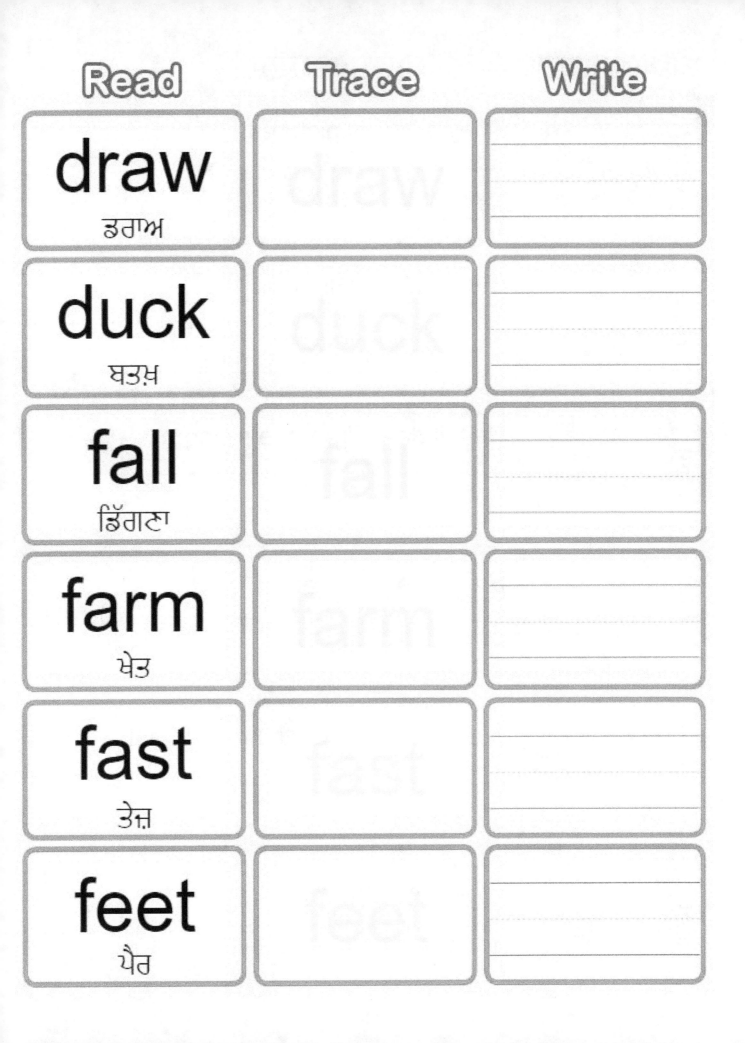

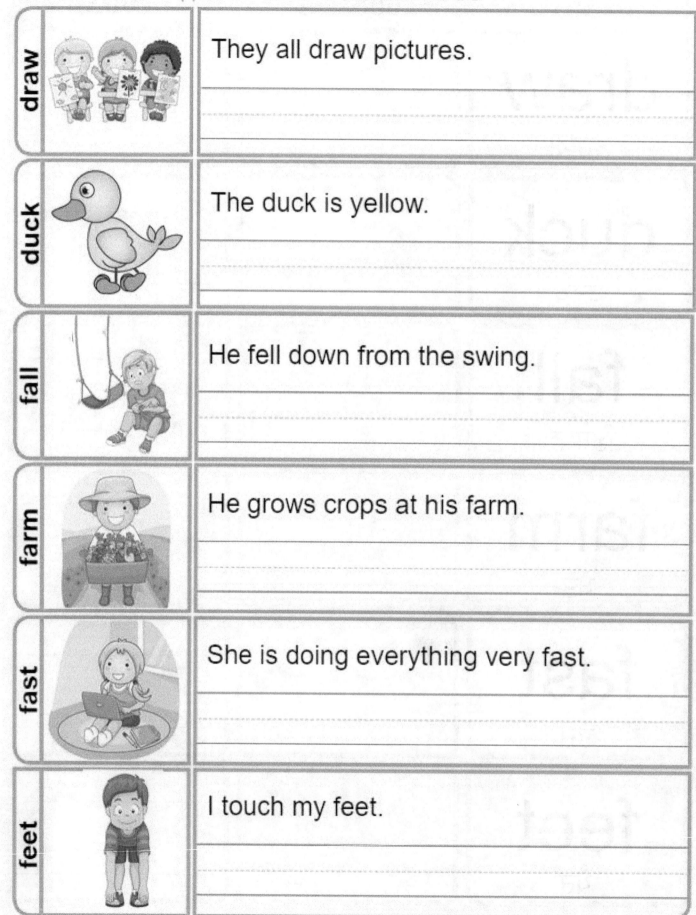

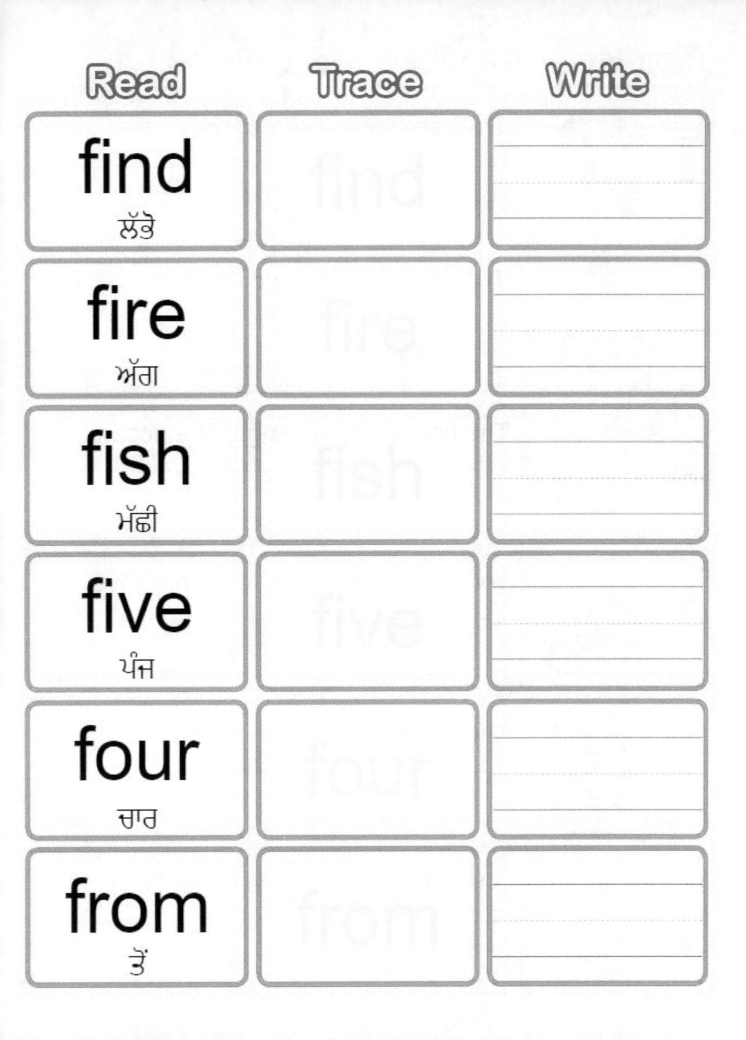

Read and write the sentence!

find	They are finding something.
fire	The fire is blazing and dangerous.
fish	The fish are swimming in the ocean.
five	You get birthday gifts for turning five.
four	The lion is turning four today.
from	She will draw a picture of her flower.

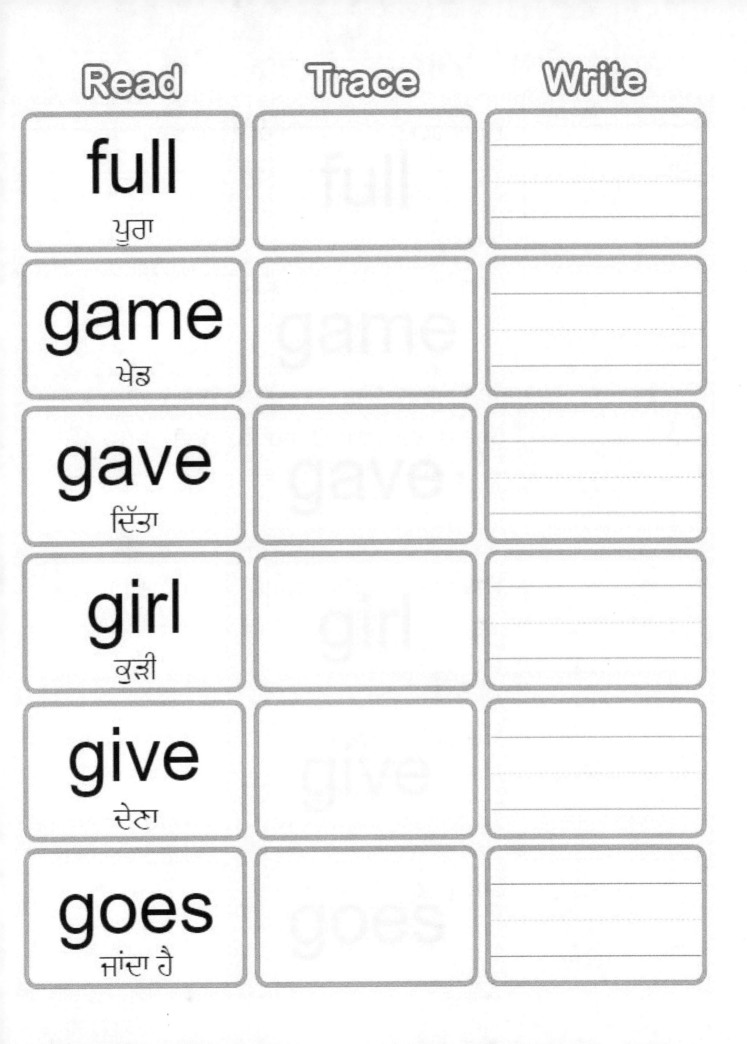

Read and write the sentence!

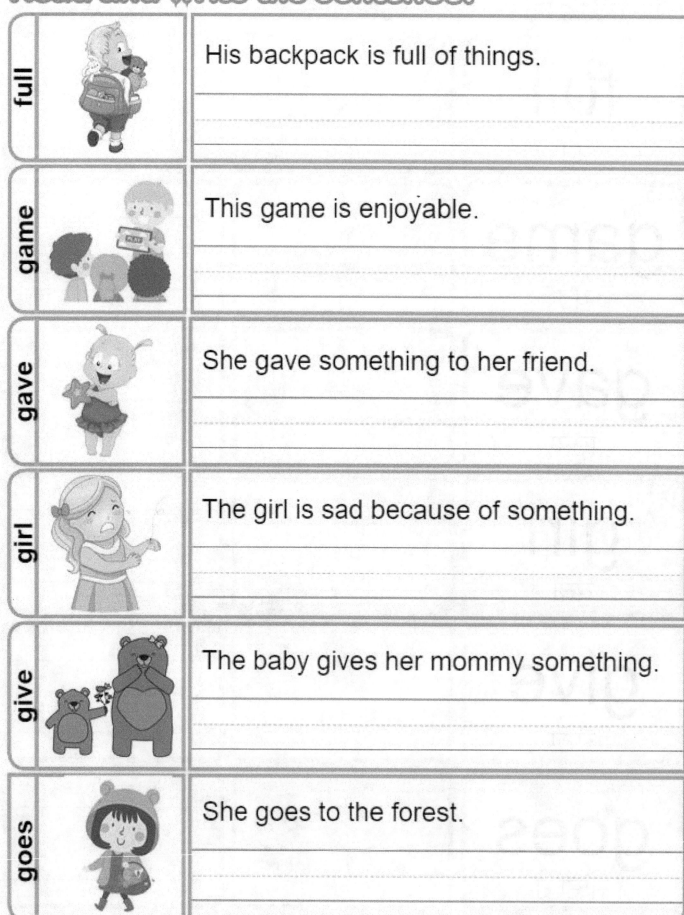

full		His backpack is full of things.
game		This game is enjoyable.
gave		She gave something to her friend.
girl		The girl is sad because of something.
give		The baby gives her mommy something.
goes		She goes to the forest.

Read	Trace	Write
good ਚੰਗਾ	good	
grow ਵਧਣ	grow	
hand ਹੱਥ	hand	
have ਹੈ	have	
head ਸਿਰ	head	
help ਮਦਦ ਕਰੋ	help	

Read and write the sentence!

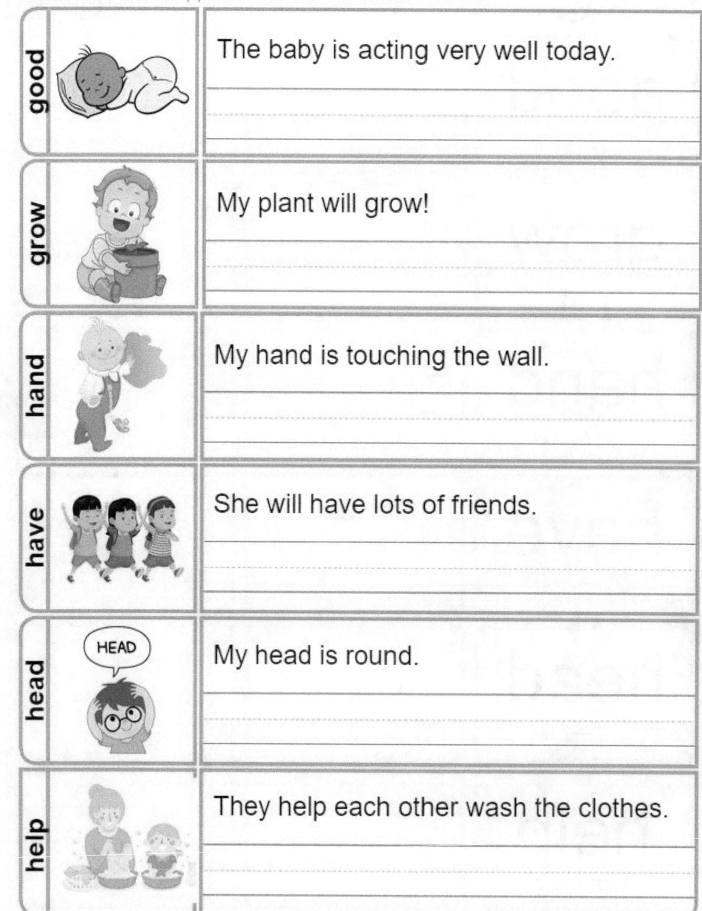

good		The baby is acting very well today.
grow		My plant will grow!
hand		My hand is touching the wall.
have		She will have lots of friends.
head		My head is round.
help		They help each other wash the clothes.

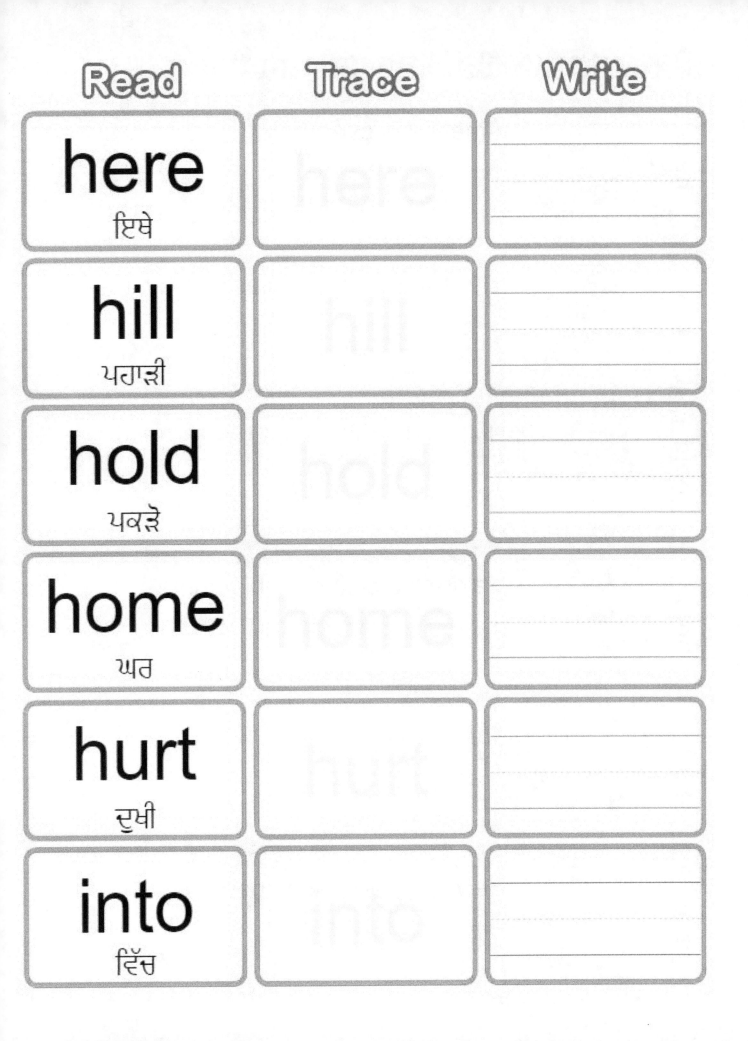

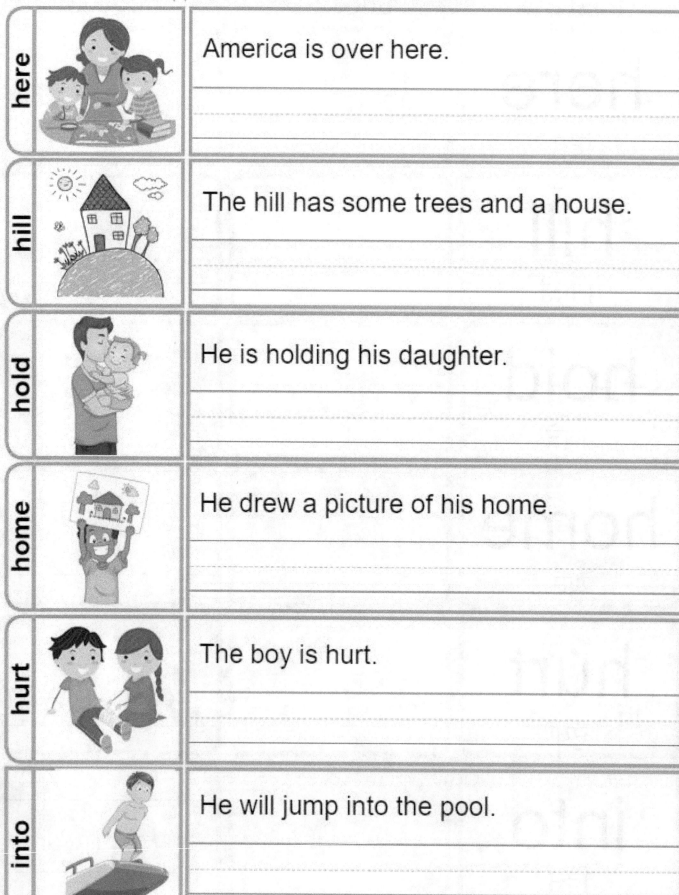

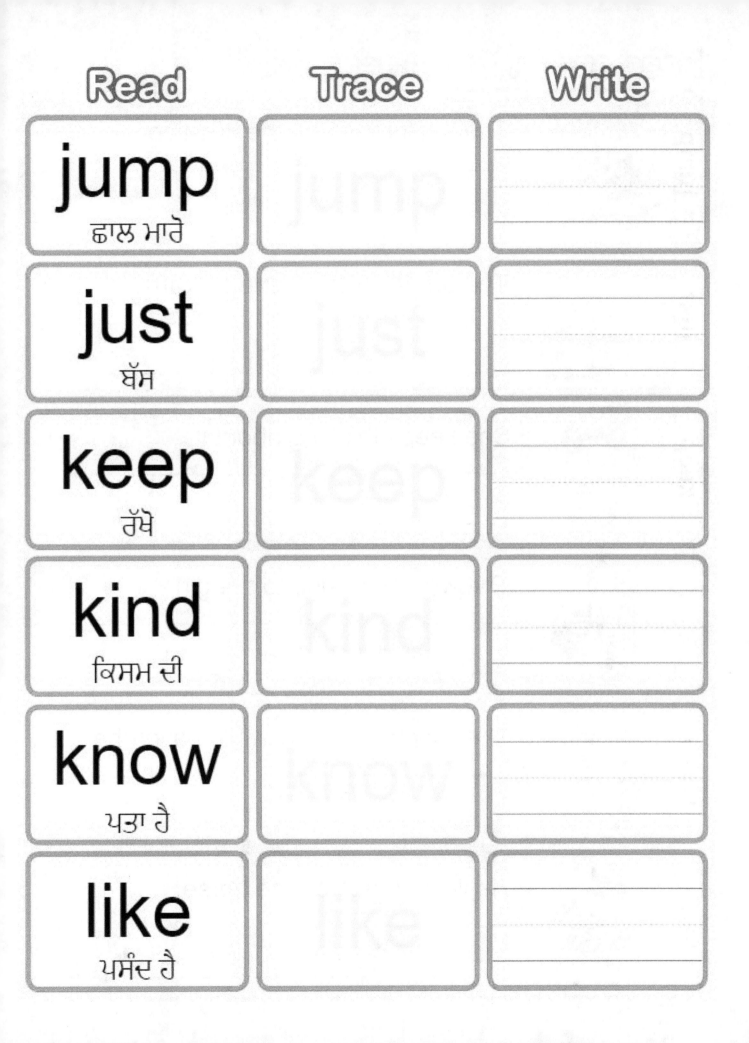

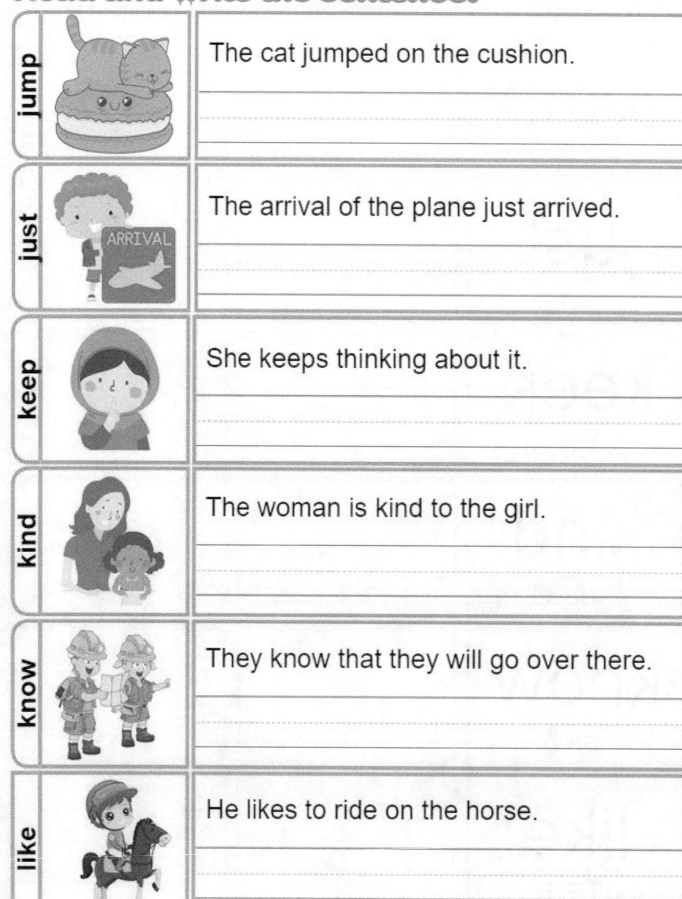

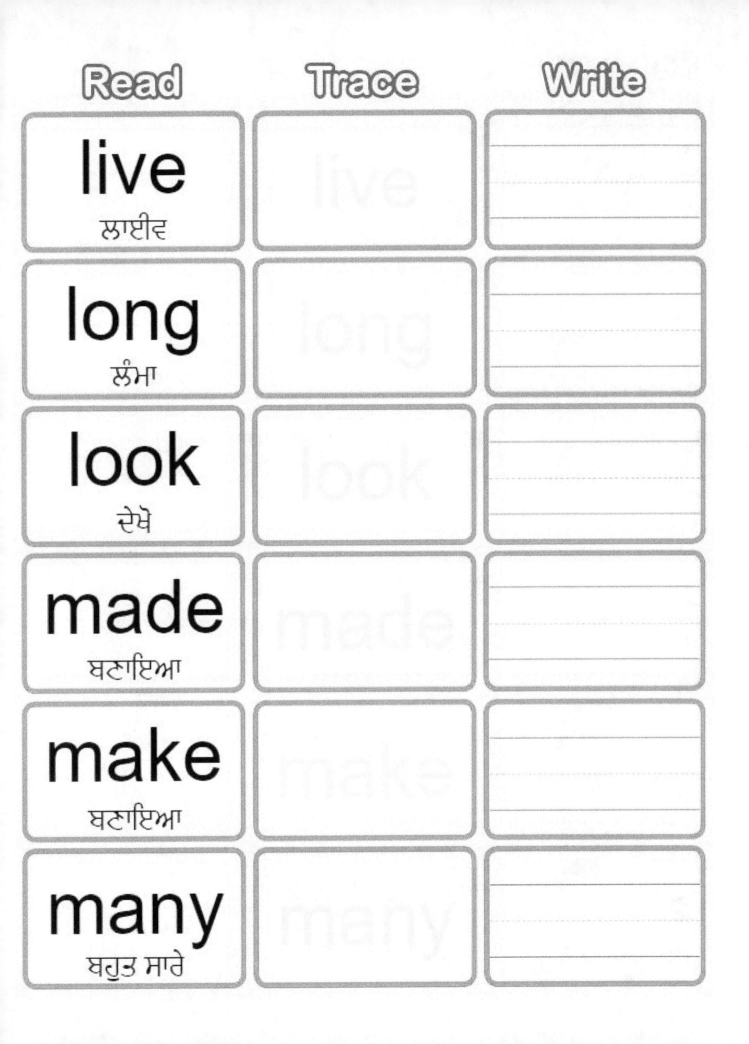

Read and write the sentence!

live	They all live together.
long	The pencil is very long.
look	They are looking at something.
made	They made a promise.
make	They are going to make something.
many	He has many shirts.

Read	Trace	Write
milk ਦੁੱਧ	milk	
much ਬਹੁਤ	much	
must ਲਾਜ਼ਮੀ ਹੈ	must	
name ਨਾਮ	name	
nest ਆਲ੍ਹਣਾ	nest	
once ਇਕ ਵਾਰ	once	

Read and write the sentence!

milk	I have milk for breakfast.
much	I like to eat this very much.
must	I must do all my homework.
name	My name is Joe.
nest	The bird has a nest.
once	He once liked to look at his computer.

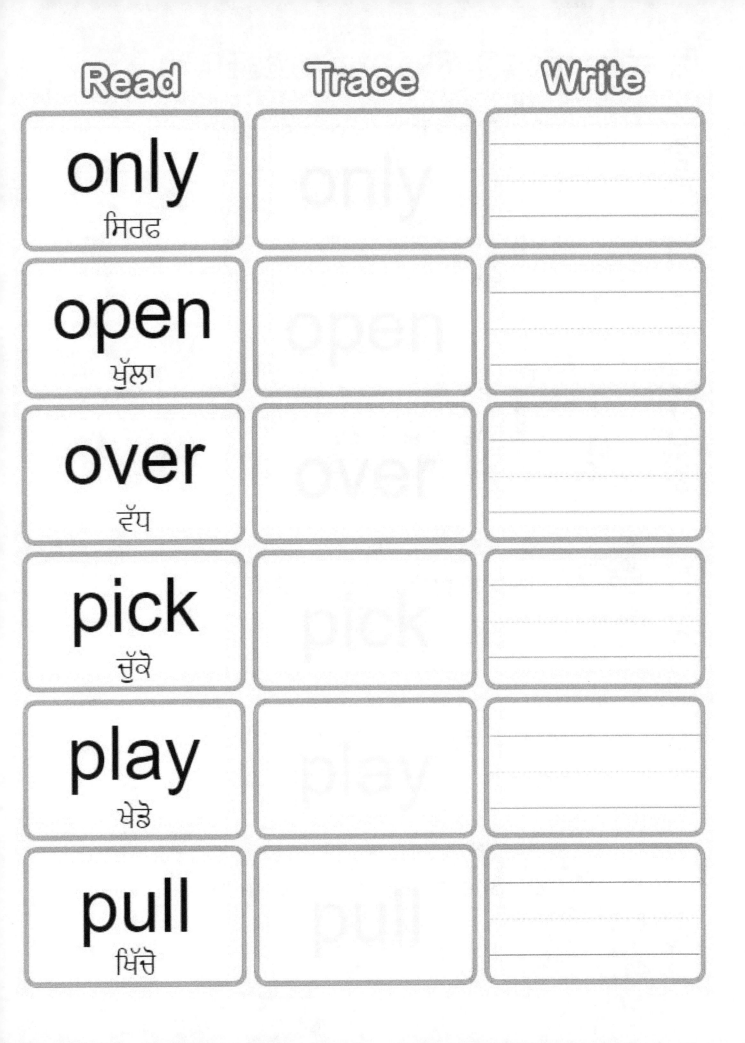

Read and write the sentence!

only		There is only one student.
open		He wants to open the door.
over		The class is over.
pick		She picked up something.
play		They like to play together.
pull		She is pulling on her friend's hair.

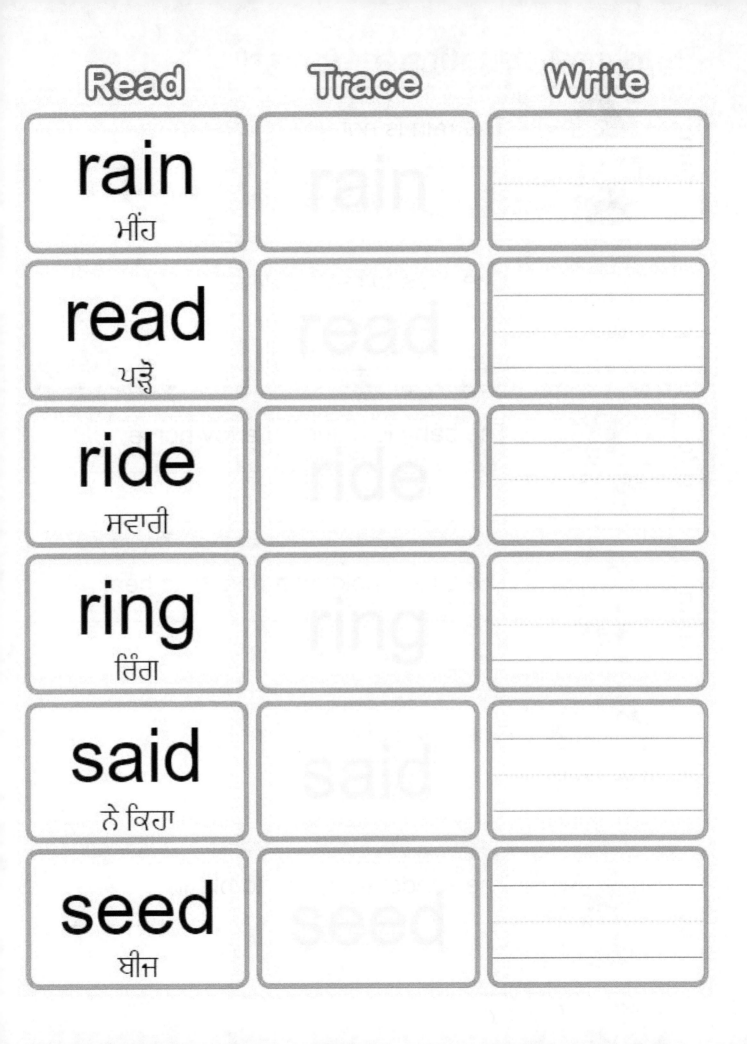

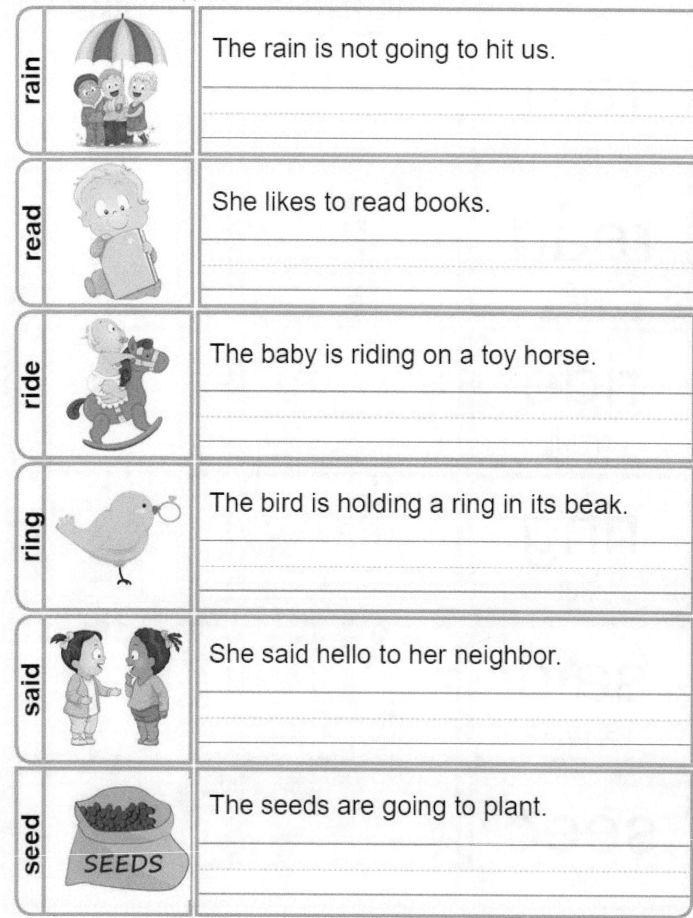

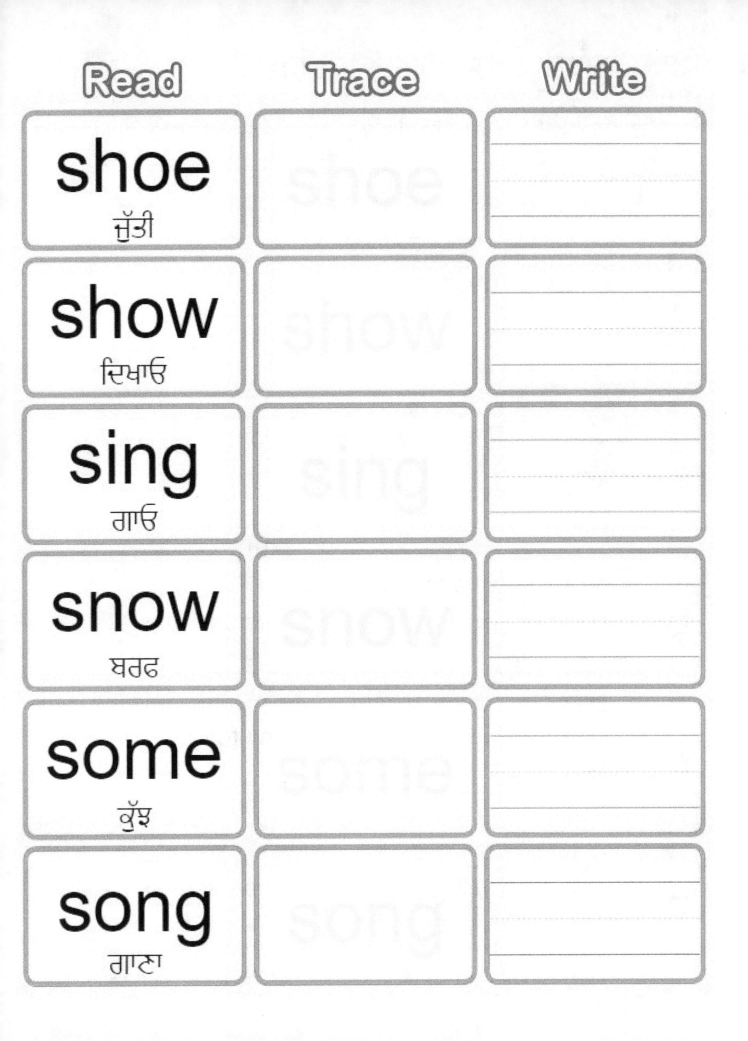

Read and write the sentence!

shoe	Her shoes are cute and purple.
show	This map shows the location.
sing	The baby can sing along.
snow	I like to play snow.
some	These are some of my toys.
song	I will sing a song in the talent show.

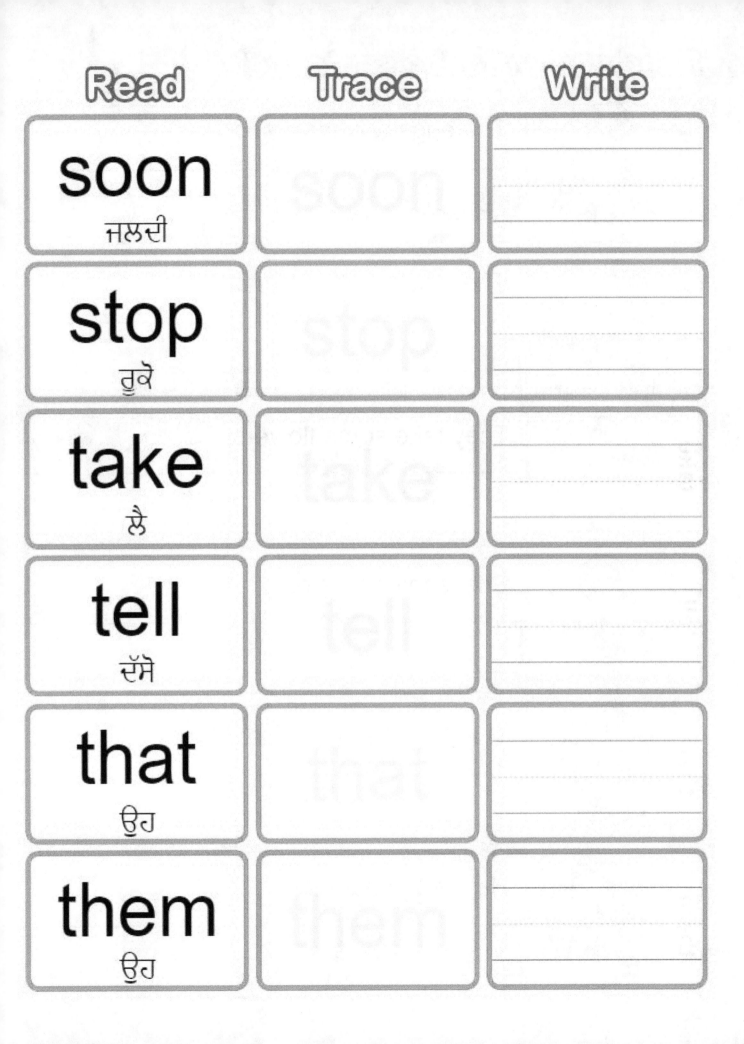

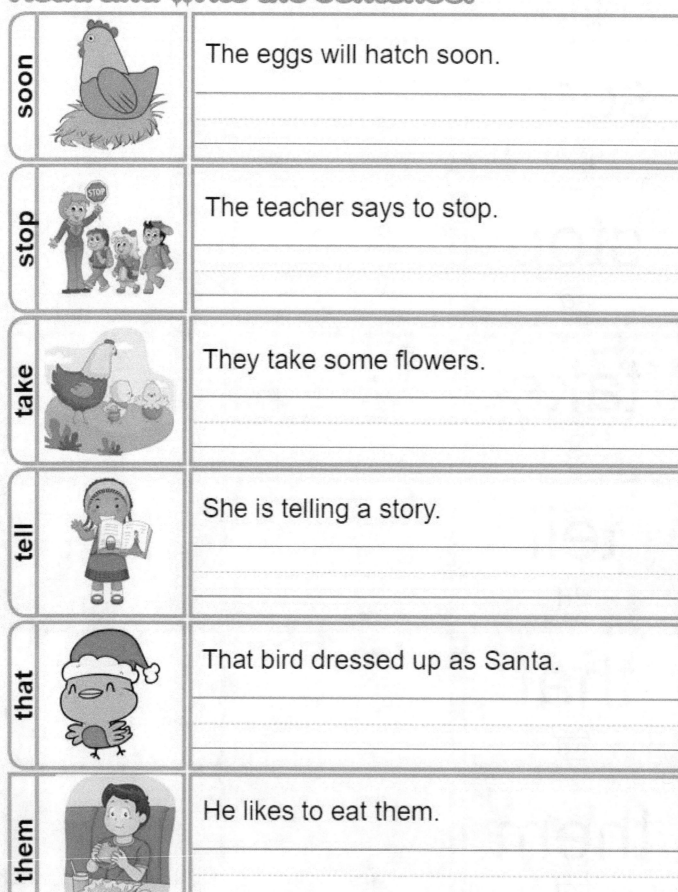

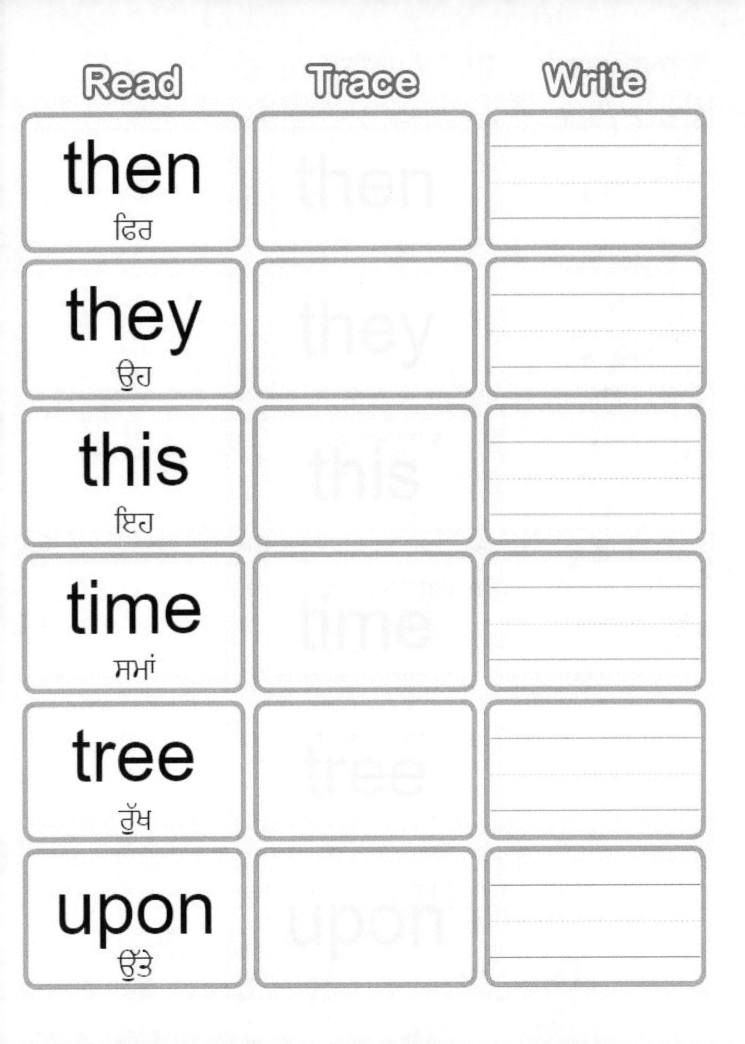

Read and write the sentence!

then		Then, I will go to bed.
they		They are running to school.
this		This is my duck.
time		The time always moves on.
tree		There are lots of green trees in the park.
upon		Once upon a time, there was a princess.

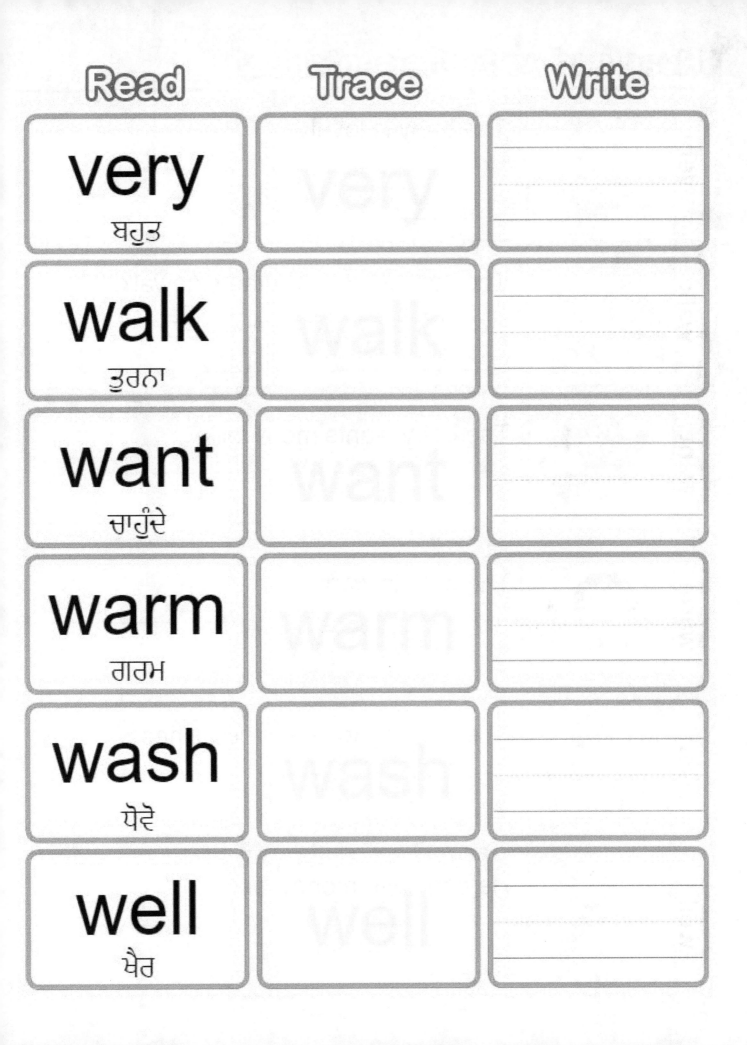

Read and write the sentence!

very		The baby is lovely.
walk		They are walking on the sidewalk.
want		The baby wants more milk.
warm		The bath is warm.
wash		She is going to wash the dishes.
well		He can save money well.

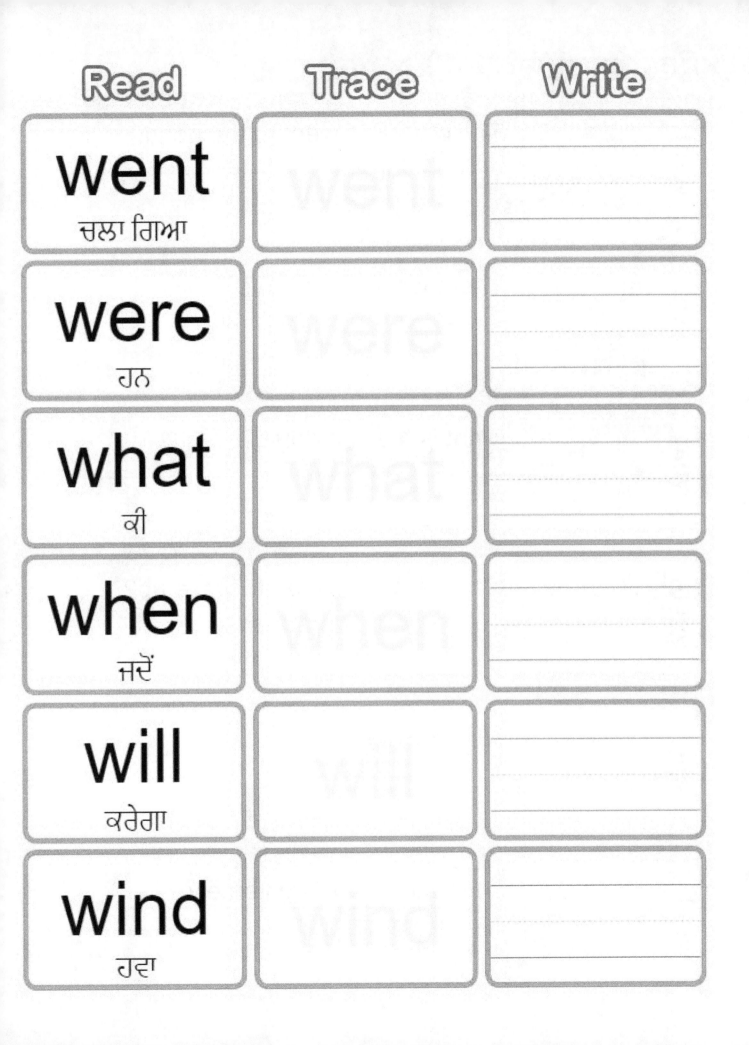

Read and write the sentence!

went		The crocodile went to the pond.
were		There were lots of toys.
what		What is the lion doing?
when		When are you going to wake up?
will		Will I get it in?
wind		The wind is blowing fiercely.

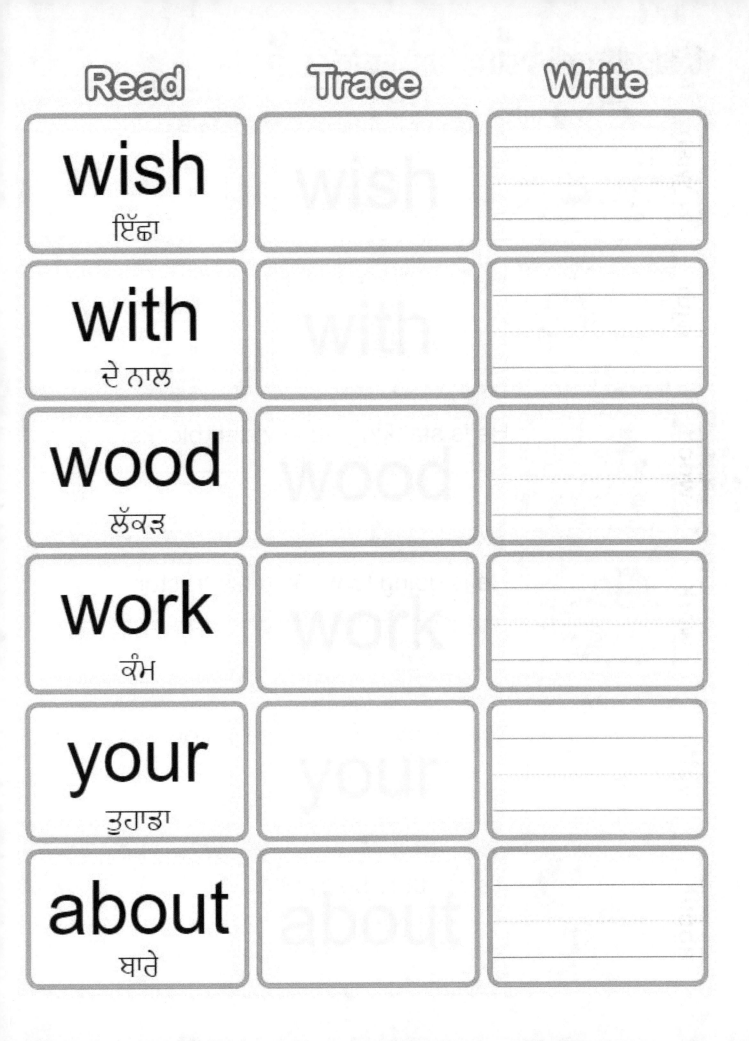

Read and write the sentence!

wish		I wish you a happy Christmas!
with		He is with his sister.
wood		He is stacking up wooden blocks.
work		He is going to work in his tractor.
your		Your baby is wearing a yellow suit.
about		It's about to be 12:30.

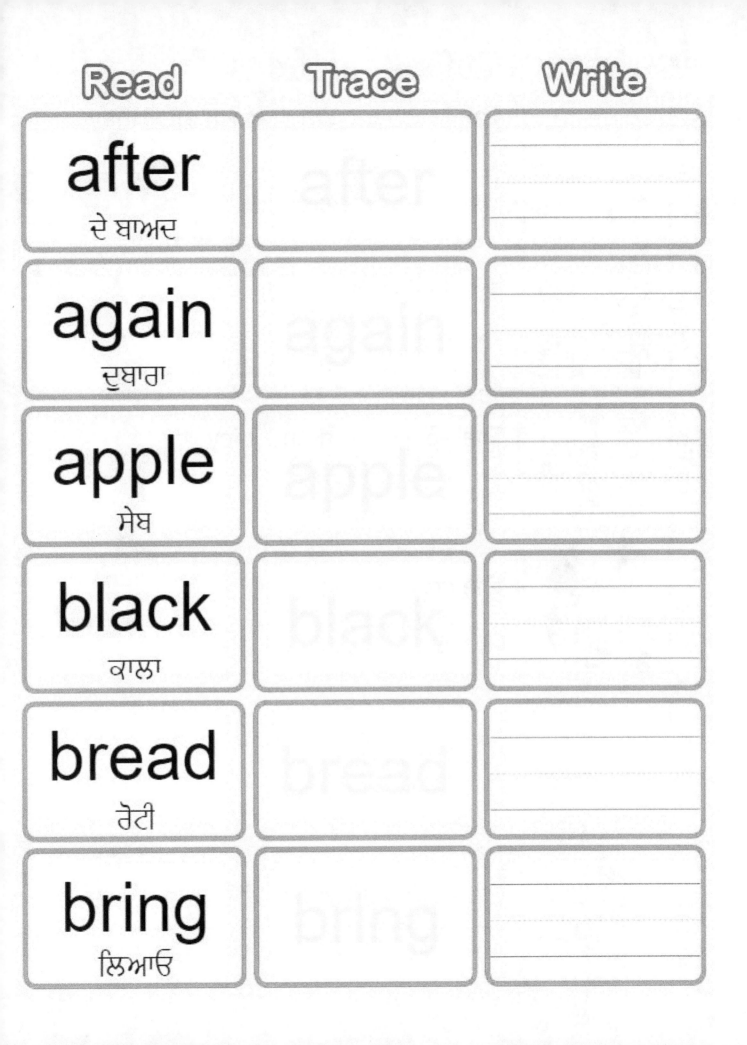

Read and write the sentence!

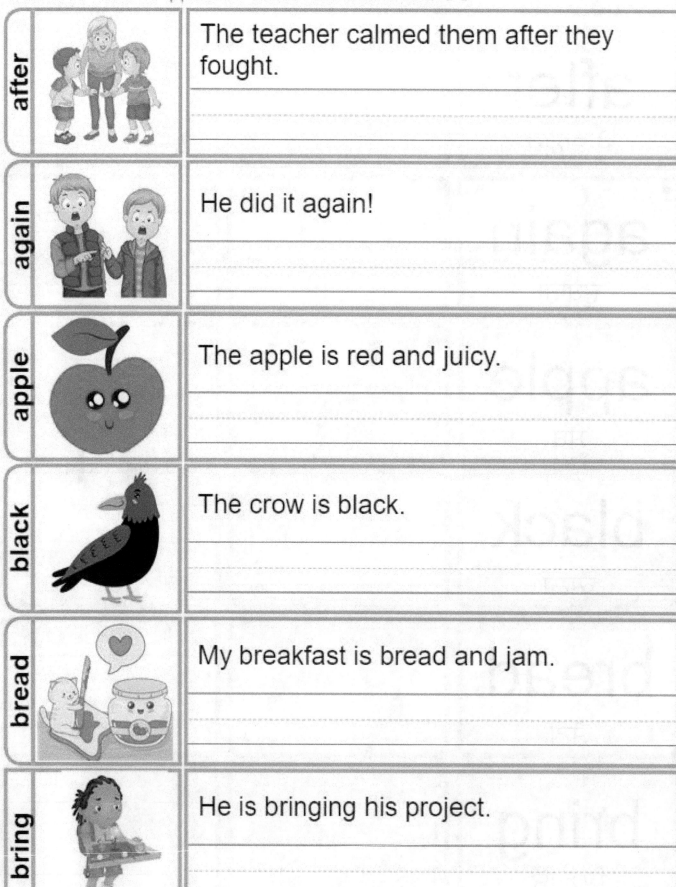

Read	Trace	Write
brown ਭੂਰਾ	brown	
carry ਲੈ	carry	
chair ਕੁਰਸੀ	chair	
clean ਸਾਫ	clean	
could ਕਰ ਸਕਦਾ ਹੈ	could	
don't ਨਾ ਕਰੋ	don't	

Read and write the sentence!

brown		Her stuffed animal is a brown bear.
carry		He is carrying a big crayon.
chair		He is sitting on his chair.
clean		He needs to clean up.
could		The baby could do push-ups.
don't		Don't do that!

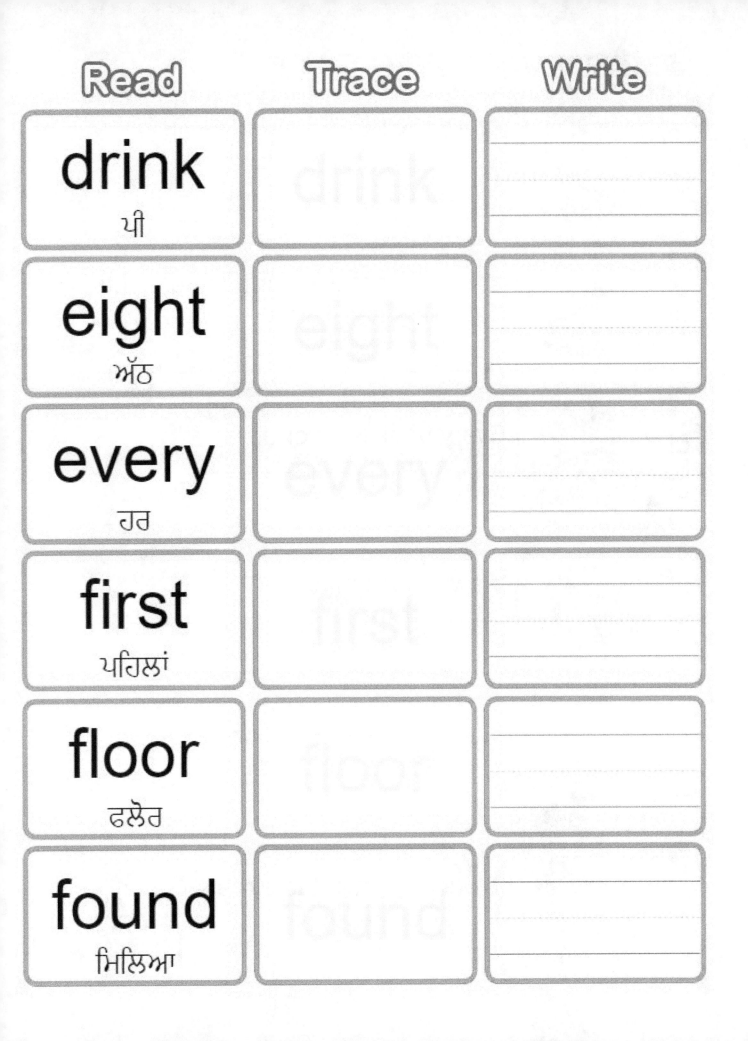

Read and write the sentence!

drink	The baby likes to drink water.
eight	You get eight gifts for turning eight!
every	Every book is colorful.
first	We won first place.
floor	She is sitting on the floor.
found	It found a hat in the streets.

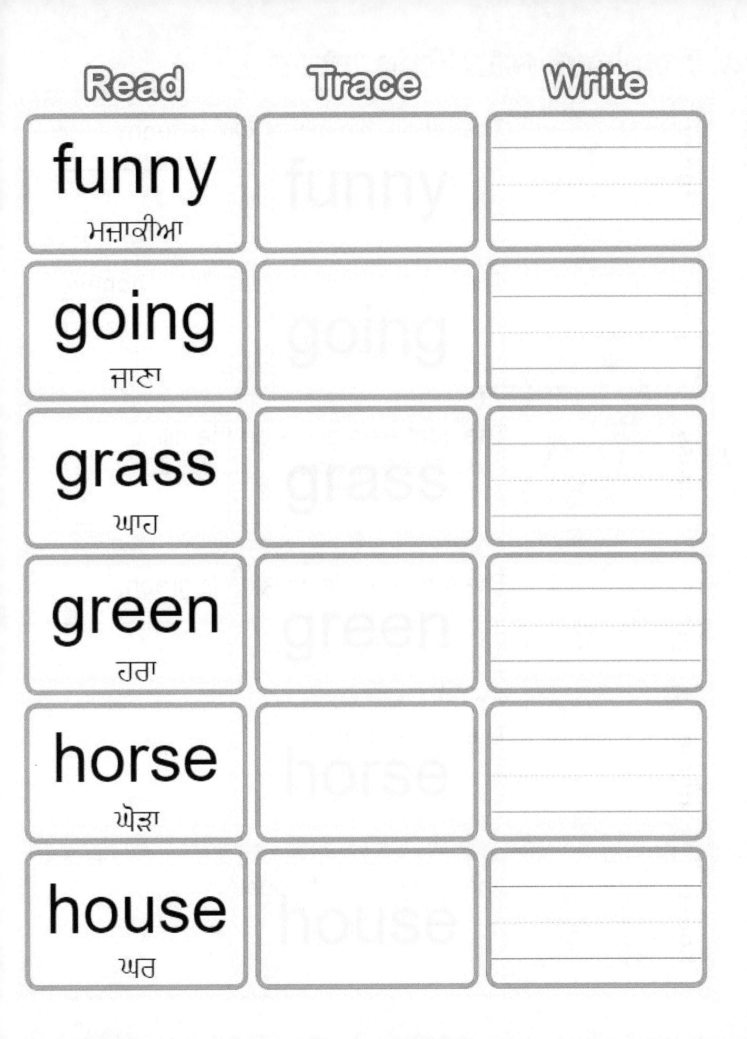

Read and write the sentence!

funny	The rabbit thinks the joke is funny.
going	The bear is going to eat all the honey.
grass	The goat eats grass on the hill.
green	The turtle that is walking is green.
horse	The horse is magical.
house	They lived in that house.

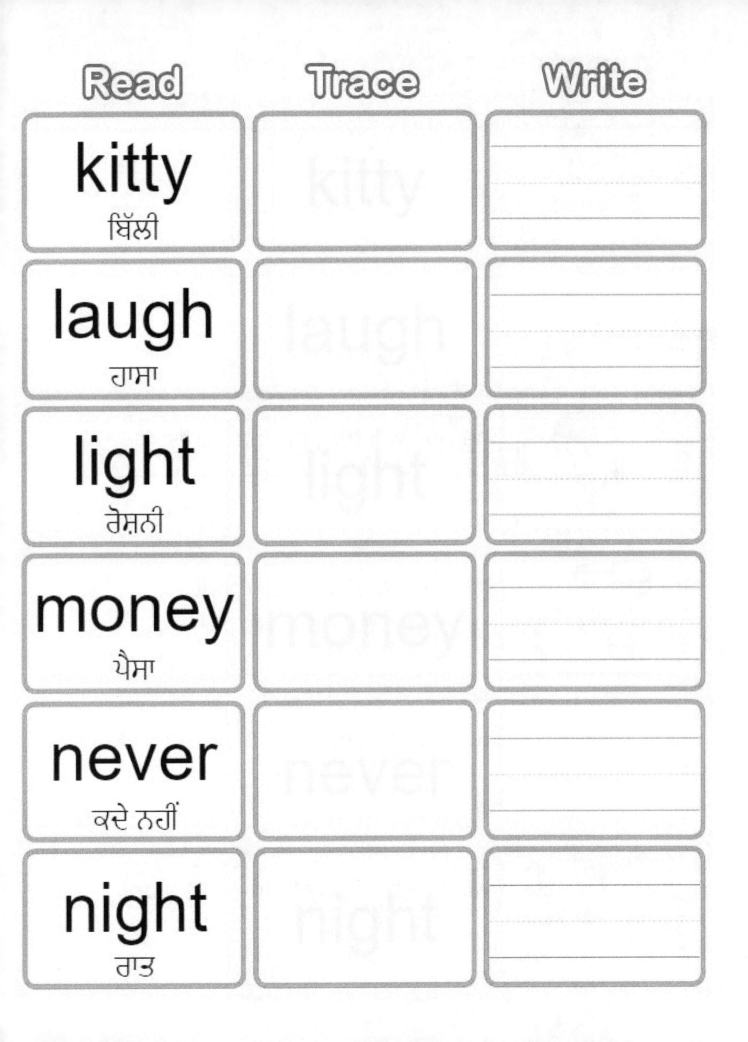

Read and write the sentence!

kitty	The kitties are charming.
laugh	They are laughing while playing.
light	The boy will turn on the lights.
money	I have earned a lot of money.
never	The bear never ate ice cream before.
night	I will sleep on my blanket at night.

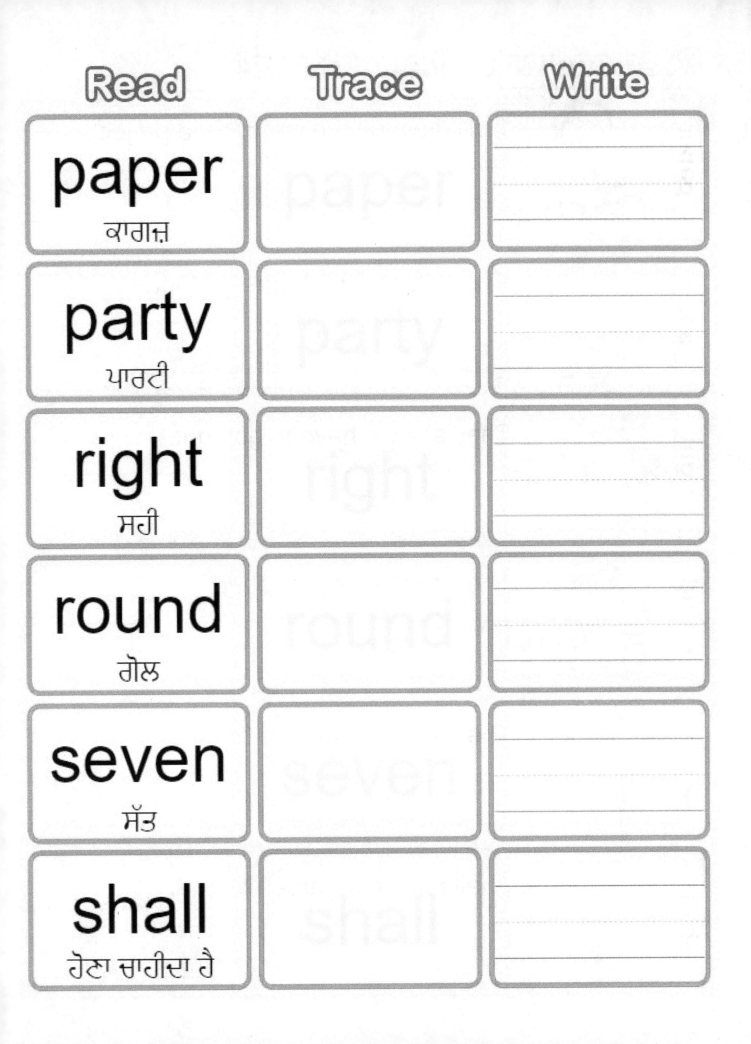

Read and write the sentence!

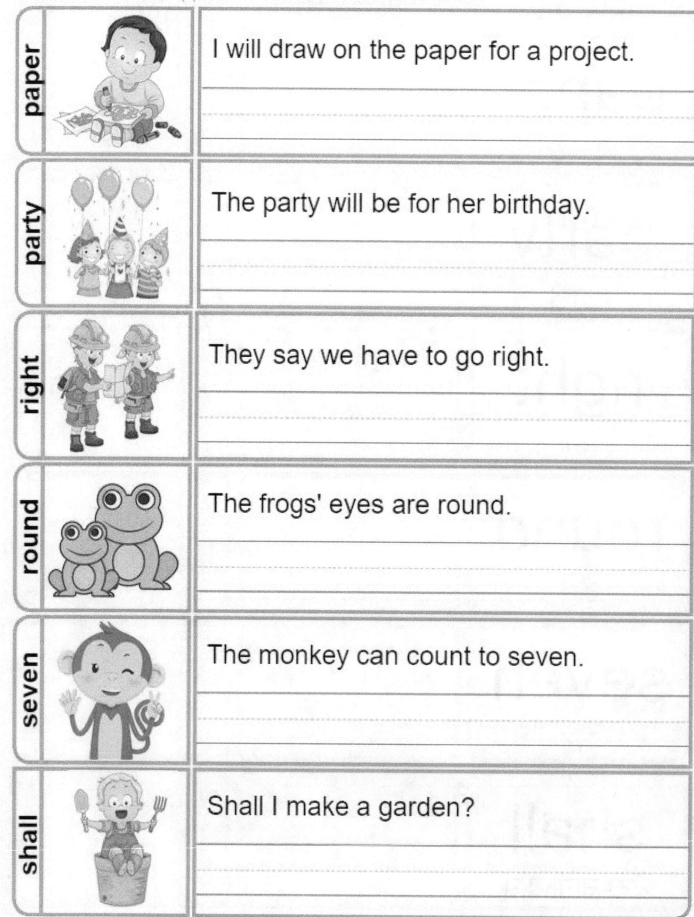

paper		I will draw on the paper for a project.
party		The party will be for her birthday.
right		They say we have to go right.
round		The frogs' eyes are round.
seven		The monkey can count to seven.
shall		Shall I make a garden?

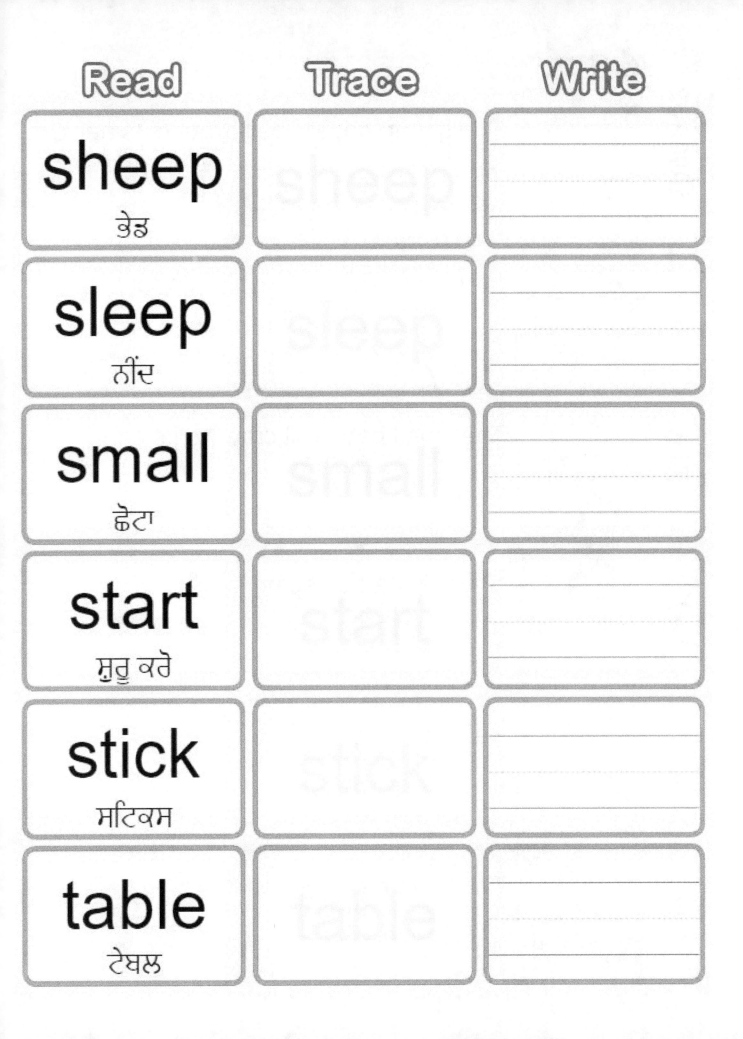

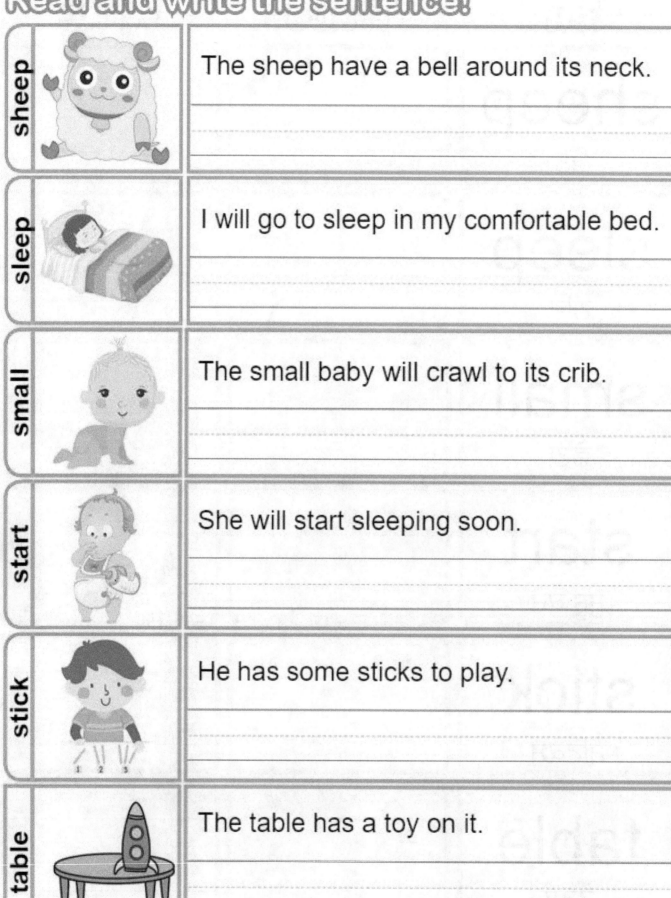

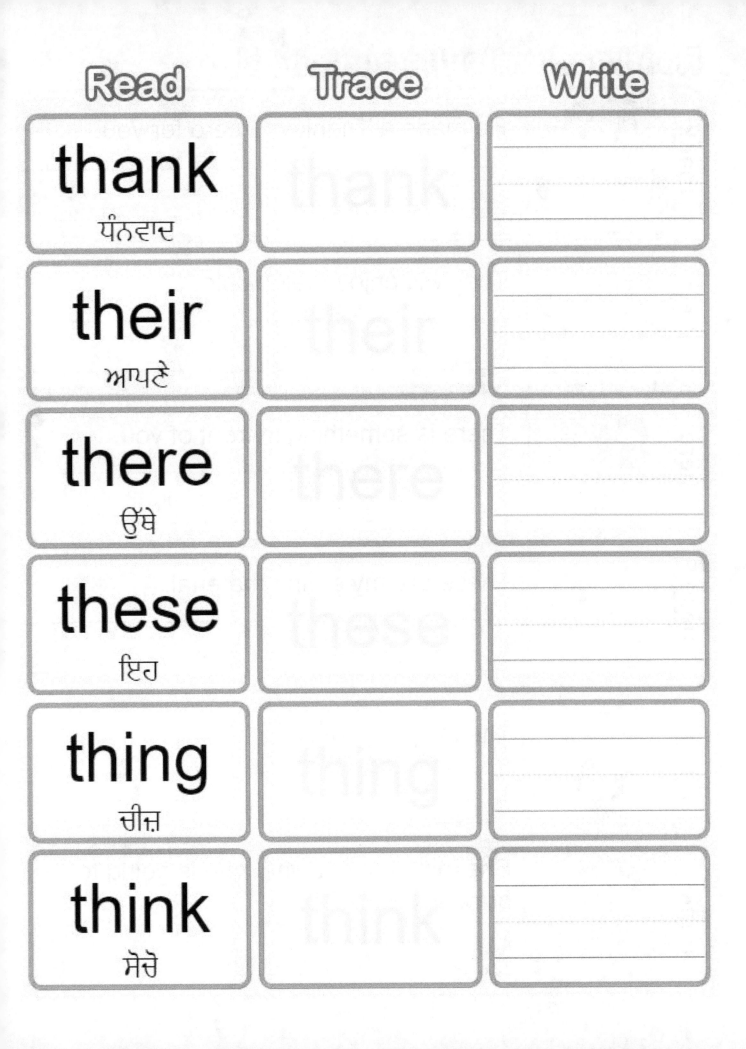

Read and write the sentence!

thank		He made a Thank you card for you.
their		They will enjoy their picnic.
there		There is something in front of you.
these		These are my eating material.
thing		The thing is broken.
think		She thinks about what she is going to draw.

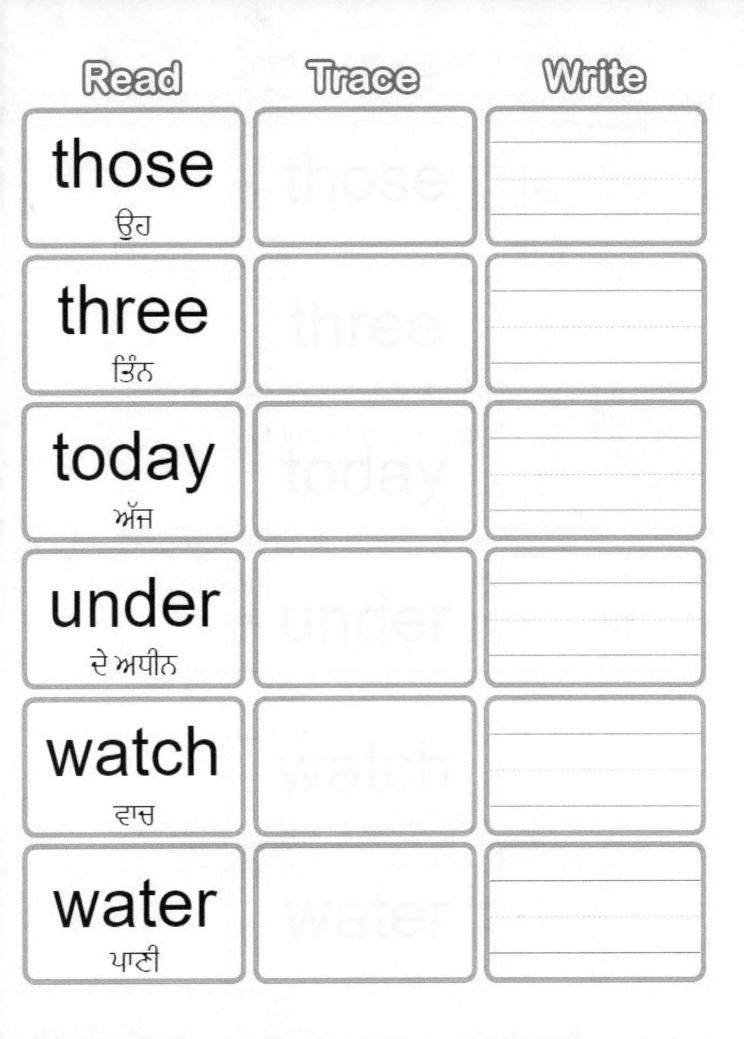

Read and write the sentence!

those		Those are mine.
three		She will turn three today.
today		Today is a beautiful day.
under		The puppy sleeps under the blanket.
watch		They both watch the video.
water		He is drinking water after a long soccer game.

Read	Trace	Write
where ਕਿੱਥੇ	where	
which ਕਿਹੜਾ	which	
white ਚਿੱਟਾ	white	
would ਹੋਵੇਗਾ	would	
write ਲਿਖੋ	write	
always ਹਮੇਸ਼ਾ	always	

Read and write the sentence!

where	Where are we?
which	The clothes which are my sisters are colorful.
white	The sheep have white wool.
would	He would tell them a story.
write	I like to write lots of stories.
always	I am always happy that it is Christmas.

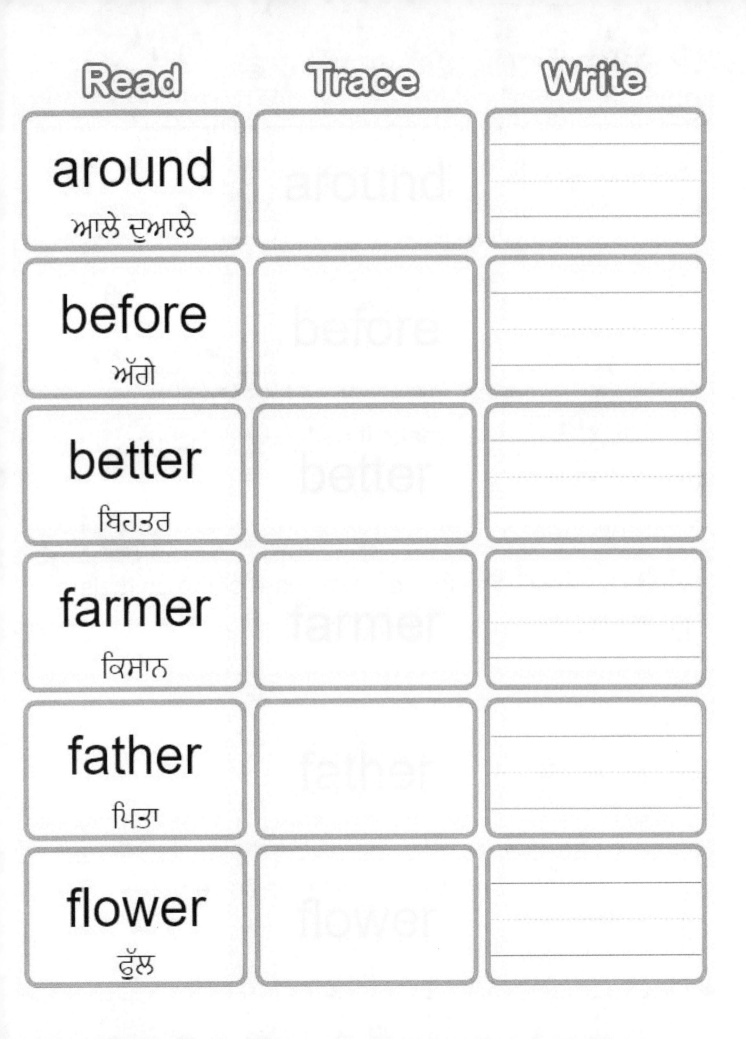

Read and write the sentence!

around		I will shuffle the shapes around.
before		Before I go to school, I kiss my mom.
better		I can make it better.
farmer		The farmer takes care of the animals.
father		My father is wearing a blue shirt.
flower		She will play with the flowers.

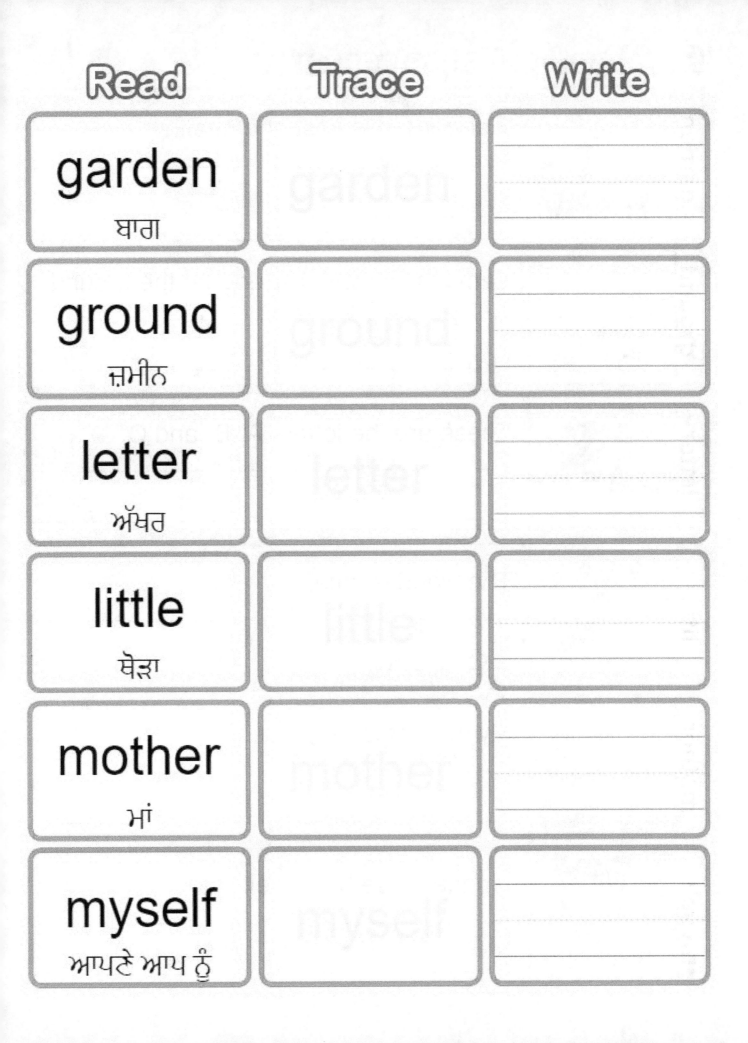

Read and write the sentence!

garden		Her garden is vast and healthy.
ground		I am playing with my dog on the ground.
letter		These are the letters A, B, and C.
little		The world is small.
mother		My mother is very nice.
myself		I made these by myself.

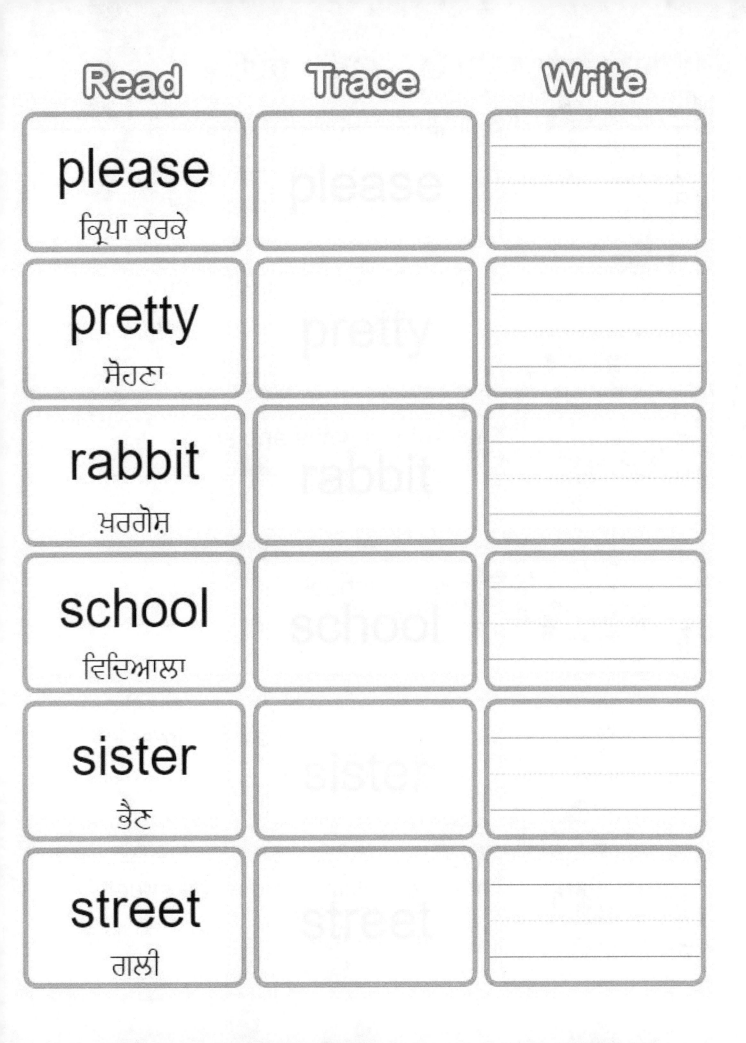

Read and write the sentence!

please		Please stop pulling my hair.
pretty		She made the cake very pretty.
rabbit		The rabbit is white and soft.
school		This is the school.
sister		My sister is wearing a pink dress.
street		They are walking across the street.

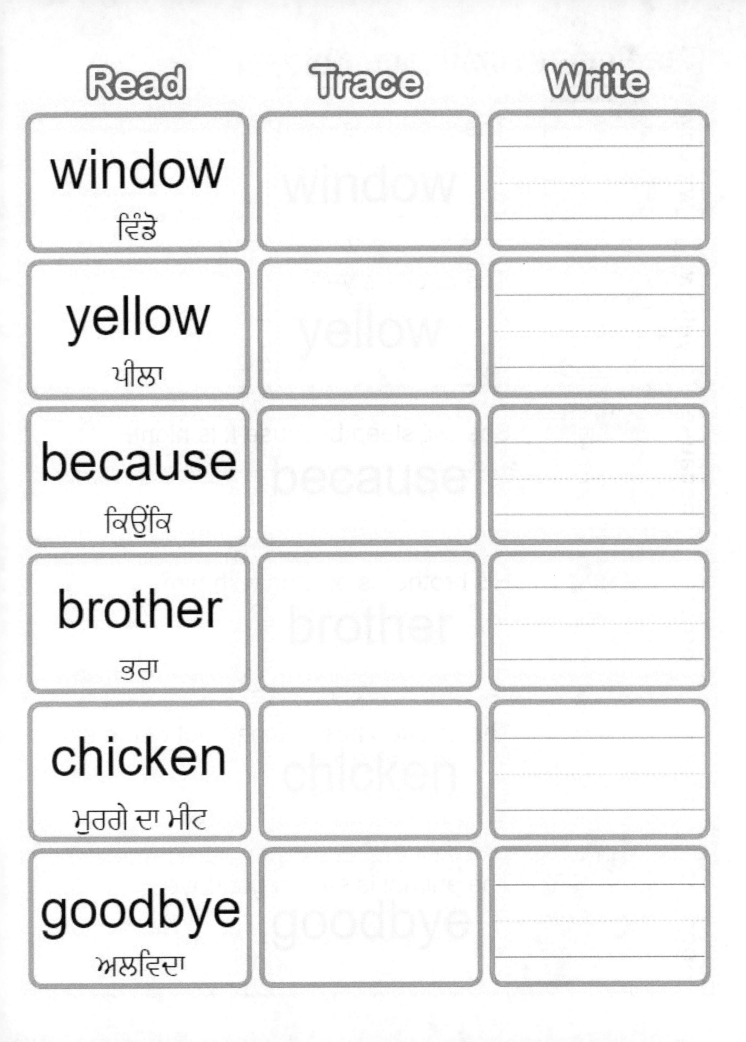

Read and write the sentence!

window		The window is open.
yellow		The ducky is yellow.
because		She will sleep because it is night.
brother		His brother is playing with him.
chicken		The chicken has hatched out of the egg.
goodbye		The animal is saying goodbye.

Read	Trace	Write
morning ਸਵੇਰ	morning	
picture ਤਸਵੀਰ	picture	
birthday ਜਨਮਦਿਨ	birthday	
children ਬੱਚੇ	children	
squirrel ਖਿਲਾਰਾ	squirrel	
together ਇਕੱਠੇ	together	

Read and write the sentence!

morning — He likes to ride his bike in the morning.

picture — He will take a picture.

birthday — Today is my birthday!

children — The children are doing something.

squirrel — The squirrel is cute.

together — They are sharing a bed together.

CPSIA information can be obtained
at www.ICGtesting.com
Printed in the USA
BVHW061037101021
618623BV00016B/1290